ILLINOIS CENTRAL COLLEGE

W9-BXD-571

A12901 379191

Withdrawn

An individual's decision to use alcohol and the frequency, quantity, and situation of such use are the result of a combination of biological and social factors. Drinking is not only a personal choice, but also a matter of custom and social behavior, and is influenced by access and economic factors, including levels of disposable income and cost of alcoholic beverages.

Until prevention efforts cease to focus narrowly on the individual and begin to adopt broader community perspectives on alcohol problems and strategies to reduce them, these efforts will fail. The author challenges the curent implicit models used in alcohol problem prevention and demonstrates an ecological perspective of the community as a complex adaptive system composed of interacting subsystems, an appreciation and understanding of which offers a new approach to the prevention of alcohol dependence and alcohol-related problems.

ALCOHOL AND THE COMMUNITY:
A SYSTEMS APPROACH TO PREVENTION

INTERNATIONAL RESEARCH MONOGRAPHS IN THE ADDICTIONS (IRMA)

Series Editor
Professor Griffith Edwards
National Addiction Centre
Institute of Psychiatry, London

A series of volumes presenting important research from major centers around the world on the basic sciences, both biological and behavioral, that have a bearing on the addictions, and also addressing the clinical and public health applications of such research. The series will cover alcohol, illicit drugs, psychotropics and tobacco, and is an important resource for clinicians, researchers and policy-makers.

Also in this series:

Cannabis and Cognitive Functioning
Nadia Solowij

ALCOHOL AND THE COMMUNITY: A SYSTEMS APPROACH TO PREVENTION

HAROLD D. HOLDER

Director and Senior Scientist, Prevention Research Center, Berkeley, California, USA

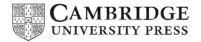

CAMBRIDGE
UNIVERSITY PRESS

HV
5035
.H65
1998

PUBLISHED BY THE PRESS SYNDICATE OF THE UNIVERSITY OF CAMBRIDGE
The Pitt Building, Trumpington Street, Cambridge CB2 1RP, United Kingdom

CAMBRIDGE UNIVERSITY PRESS
The Edinburgh Building, Cambridge CB2 2RU, United Kingdom
40 West 20th Street, New York, NY 10011-4211, USA
10 Stamford Road, Oakleigh, Melbourne 3166, Australia

© Harold D. Holder 1998

This book is in copyright. Subject to statutory exception
and to the provisions of relevant collective licensing agreements,
no reproduction of any part may take place without
the written permission of Cambridge University Press.

First published 1998

Printed in the United Kingdom at the University Press, Cambridge

Typset in Times 10/13 pt [VN]

A catalogue record for this book is available from the British Library

Library of Congress Cataloguing in Publication data

Holder, Harold D.
    Alcohol and the community: a systems approach to prevention/
Harold D. Holder
        p.   cm. – (International research monographs in the
additions
    ISBN 0 521 59187 2 (hardcover)
    1. Alcoholism – Social aspects.   2. Alcoholism – Prevention.
I. Title.   II. Series.
HV5035.H65   1998
362.292'7–dc21   97–20455 CIP

This book is dedicated to my father, Benjamin Solomon Holder, whose earliest teaching to his young son was about the naturalness of the world. I learned the language and concepts of complex adaptive systems later in life but my appreciation of such systems is rooted in my father's perspective.

Contents

Series editor's preface

Alcohol issues are a cause today for intense public health concern in most countries of the world. That assertion is valid for rich nations whose encounters with drink have long histories, and poorer regions where the adverse consequences of alcohol may begin to threaten national development.

Within the modern Public Health perspective, alcohol, the commodity itself, is an issue of concern as well as the problems which drinking generates. The reason for taking this position is the overwhelming strength of the research evidence showing that the more an individual drinks, the greater the risk of that person sustaining alcohol-related harm. Similarly, the higher the national per capita alcohol consumption, the greater will be the alcohol-related burden of costs and damage for that society.

The Public Health perspective is also illuminated by studies which demonstrate the immense variety in types and degree of the problems which can be caused by drinking. The concerns must be with the sum of small problems as well as with large problems, with harm done to the family or bystander as well as the direct consequences for the drinker themselves, with acute mishaps as well as chronic illness, and with the problems which occur in the social as well as the medical domain. These matters cannot be tidied away by directing our responses solely at 'the alcoholic'.

Dr Harold Holder's analysis brilliantly exemplifies this perspective. While not discounting the background importance of national alcohol policy responses, he offers an analysis at the level of local community. His essential argument is that to deal effectively with control over access to alcohol and to the multifarious problems engendered by alcohol, multiple actions will be needed by many types of community actor. He offers an incisive view on how that essentially ecological perspective is to be systemised.

This is a book which advances theory and sets research agendas, but at the same time it speaks practically to front-line alcohol issues within our communities, how to prevent the related suffering and costs, and how to save lives. Its author is American, but its messages are of wide international applicability.

Harold Holder enjoys great esteem as a distinguished researcher in this field. In this innovative text he demonstrates his capacity to make scientific analysis relevant at the street corner, both actual and metaphorical.

Griffith Edwards
National Addiction Centre
London, February 1997

Acknowledgements

Many have contributed to this book. I wish to acknowledge the hard work and dedication of Janet Jester in preparing multiple versions of this manuscript and its many drawings and tables. My co-workers with *SimCom* over the years were my worthy tutors in developing operational computer models. Special appreciation must be given to Jim Blose who worked along side me for over ten years through various versions of *SimCom*. In recent years, the interest and energy of Barry Kibel and Will Miner expanded the model with further complexity, as well as enhanced user support and careful documentation. Robert Reynolds whose vision about science-based technology to aid alcohol prevention was an inspiration for computer modeling and for this book. Thanks to all of you and to others who contributed but were not named here.

I want to express appreciation to the Santa Fe Institute (SFI), Santa Fe, New Mexico (USA), for the intellectual support and stimulation concerning complex adaptive systems and for providing lodging during two extended visits during which time I wrote this book. SFI is fulfilling a critical nexus for cross-discipline exchange concerning chaos theory and adaptive systems.

Harold D. Holder

1
The community system of alcohol use and alcohol problems

Introduction

Joseph Townsend lives in Great Britain in the large metropolitan area of Birmingham. Concerned about the number of street people in his downtown neighborhood who were regularly intoxicated, Joseph organized his neighbors and many local shops to set up a storefront recovery center where alcohol-dependent people could get counseling and where meetings of self-help groups, e.g., Alcoholics Anonymous, could be held. The storefront recovery center was a big success, with many clients coming and going every day. After the center had been operating successfully for six months, Joseph noticed, during his regular walks through his neighborhood, that the number of people intoxicated on the street had not decreased. In fact, there appeared to be many more now than before. "How could this be," he wondered, "after all the work we have done?"

In another community, Silver City, a small multi-ethnic town in New Mexico (USA), Mary and Charles Lopez, parents of two children, 15 and 18 years old, were concerned about the amount of drinking by local young people. They were fearful that their daughter and son might drink, and they were concerned about the risk of harm to their children and others in their community as a result of teenage drinking. Other parents joined them in assisting the local schools to adopt a health curriculum that informed young people about the risks of alcohol and other drugs. The school curriculum was widely and effectively implemented, and was popularly received by the community. About a year later, four honor-roll students were killed during a "joy ride" in a family automobile. The 17–year-old driver had a blood alcohol level of 0.15%, well over the legal limit. In covering the tragic deaths, the local paper noted that, according to a recent survey, self-reported alcohol use among high school students was at an all-time high. It also reported that all the young people in the car had been drinking, and that they had just left a party where a keg of beer was available, permitting unlimited drinking.

In Vancouver, British Columbia (western Canada), scientists were working on a longitudinal research project to determine the characteristics of children most at risk for early alcohol use and subsequent high-volume, dependent use. The scientists developed a set of factors that statistically predicted which children would be most likely to engage in experimental drinking. Such factors as hyperactivity, shyness, loneliness, and family history of problem drinking (possibly suggesting a genetic component to risk) were identified. As a result of their success in isolating these factors, the scientists received much attention from other researchers. Working with the local school district, they obtained federal government funds for a research demonstration project. They used the grant funds to establish and evaluate a program to identify 6– to 8–year-old children at risk, and to counsel their families. Students were assigned randomly to treatment groups, in which children at risk were identified and their families were counseled, and to control groups, which received no intervention. At the end of the ten-year study, drinking rates in the treatment group were lower than would be expected based on published reports of alcohol use in other, similar school populations. However, the control group's drinking rates also were lower than expected. The scientists published a set of scholarly papers reporting statistically significant differences between the treatment and control groups in such measures as age of initiation and drinking level. However, overall rates of drinking and driving crashes, and alcohol-related violent events among young people in the community were at their highest levels in ten years. The school superintendent, who was an enthusiastic supporter of the early identification and counseling program, wondered what had gone wrong.

In Perth, Australia, a community coalition of concerned citizens received a grant from a private foundation to plan a prevention effort against alcohol and drug abuse. The community had a high rate of alcohol-related problems and illicit drug use, so local leaders were enthusiastic about a community-wide prevention effort. At the end of the one-year planning period, a community-wide coalition of leading civic organizations, religious groups, and businesses had been organized, and the coalition had prepared a well-written plan for a long-term prevention public education campaign. As a result, the foundation gave the community an additional three-year grant to implement the full prevention program. Using foundation funds, the community hired full-time staff, established program offices in a visible location downtown, and invited additional organizations and community leaders to participate. The program initiated a series of professionally planned media campaigns to inform everyone in the community about the problem of alcohol and drug abuse. Large numbers of brochures and posters were printed, and television and radio time, and newspaper space were purchased. Novel public information techniques were used, such as messages on grocery bags, and on free balloons and candy. Messages warned about the dangers of heavy alcohol use and the community's intolerance of illicit drug use. People were impressed with the high quality of the media campaign, and it was well received. Families and young people were organized into support groups to assist the campaign. In the second year of the program, the media campaign included a week-long community forum and celebration, complete with alcohol-free events and professional musical entertainment. Media coverage of the coalition and its activities was extensive. The coalition and community support groups against alcohol and drug abuse increased in size. At the end of the program's third year, an outside university research group conducted an independent evaluation of the program. They found high community awareness, support, and participation in the campaign. However, when the researchers compared recently collected outcome data with baseline data collected before the campaign, they found no changes in the rates of alcohol-related problems or self-reported drug use. The community leaders and the foundation were displeased. The foundation refused to release the findings. The community leaders dismissed the results as irrelevant, because everyone in the community was happy with the program.

In communities throughout the world, people are concerned about drinking by young people, drinking and driving, alcohol dependency, drinking at the workplace, and accidental injuries, accidental deaths, and violence resulting from alcohol use. These health, economic, and social problems to which alcohol can significantly contribute are what we refer to in this book as "alcohol-involved problems." In the stories above, only the names and locations have been changed. These accounts illustrate the difficulties commonly experienced by communities worldwide in their efforts to prevent alcohol-involved problems.

Alcohol abuse has most often been viewed as a problem involving drunks and alcoholics – individuals whose heavy use of alcohol is regular (usually daily) and involves binge drinking and drunkenness. Prevention of alcohol-involved problems most often has focused on individual decision-making or compulsion to drink. However, such approaches to alcohol-abuse prevention fail to take into account many factors surrounding patterns of alcohol use and alcohol-involved problems. In reality, we are creatures of our cultural and economic environments, which influence us, and which we influence in turn. We are connected to other people, and our actions and reactions cause actions and reactions in others. We can use alcoholic beverages to our own advantage, or disadvantage, or to the disadvantage of those around us. An individual's decision to use alcohol, and the frequency, quantity, and situation of individual alcohol use are the result of a combination of biological and social factors, including physiology, personality, and parental behavior (what one saw as a child). What one's friends and relatives do, and what one believes to be socially expected, as well as such tangible factors as alcohol availability, how much money one has to spend, and the cost of alcoholic beverages are relative to the decision.

This book's thesis is that until prevention efforts cease to focus narrowly on individual alcoholism and begin to adopt broader perspectives on alcohol-involved problems and strategies to reduce them, the experiences described at the start of this chapter will be repeated over and over. Prevention efforts that focus only on alcoholism overlook the general misuse of alcohol and the use of alcoholic beverages in high-risk situations, such as driving or swimming. In addition, efforts that target only individuals ignore the routine social and economic context in which drinking occurs in almost every industrialized society. Drinking is not only a personal choice, but also a matter of custom and social behavior. It is influenced by disposable income, and by the availability and cost of alcoholic beverages. In traditional approaches, the well-intentioned people who introduce prevention programs into communities have rarely considered community settings as adaptive, dynamic systems – complex arrangements with parts that interact and change over time, often in unexpected ways.

The purpose of this book is to challenge the current implicit models used in alcohol problem prevention and to offer a perspective of the community as a complex adaptive system. Appreciating, understanding, and intervening in the community system is the frontier for alcohol problem prevention in the 21st century.

Heritage of the dynamic community system

All ideas have debts to those who established earlier intellectual foundations. The community perspective as a complex adaptive system follows earlier work in community psychology, general systems theory, and community-based prevention in alcohol and other drug abuse.

Community psychologists following the lead of social psychology and sociologists have for a number of years called for a consideration of the individual within the social environment in designing prevention. Lewin (1947), who introduced the construct of field theory (borrowed from physics) into psychology, laid down the principle of individual and environmental interaction. Sarason (1974) described the community as containing a variety of institutions which are formally and informally related to each other. Seidman (1988) in describing a theory of social interaction for community psychology emphasized ongoing transactions and social relationships between subsystems as well as between-system interactions. Kelly and his colleagues (Kelly et al., 1988; Kelly, 1990) have established principles for conducting prevention research in the community with a focus on community ecology.

The general systems approach to complex organizations (physical sciences, and social and behavioral sciences) defined the principles of self-organization, adaptation, and feedback across intellectual disciplines. See, for example, the description by Mitroff & Sagasti (1973) of general systems theory and complex decision-systems. Churchman (1979) and Ackoff & Emery (1972) described the elements of purposeful systems which use internal structure as well as interaction with the larger environment to survive and adapt.

There exists a long history of community-based prevention efforts for alcohol-involved problems. See reviews by Holder (1992) and Giesbrecht (1993). An example of community prevention efforts designed to alter community structures and not a target group of high-risk individuals is provided by Casswell & Gilmore (1989) in New Zealand, Stout (1992) in Rhode Island, USA, and Holmila (1997) in Finland. The community effort in Ontario, Canada, described by Giesbrecht & Pederson (1991) illustrates a mixed strategy targeting a high-risk drinking group and structural changes.

This book has an intellectual debt to such foundations. However, the concepts to be presented do represent a radical departure from most community-based prevention as practiced throughout the world currently. The complex adaptive systems perspective is not a simple extension of earlier intellectual work as the next chapter will illustrate.

Complexity, chaos, and self-adaptive systems

To understand how the perspective on alcohol-involved problems presented in this book differs from traditional perspectives, it is necessary to understand a bit about traditional Western scientific approaches – in particular, the differences between reductionist and holistic approaches to science, and between deterministic and probabilistic explanations of phenomena.

Western approaches to science and understanding have 2000–year-old roots in the writings of Aristotle, whose logical rules of reasoning (rules of valid inference) established the framework for systematic and scientific thinking since his time. These logical rules of reasoning include *induction*, by which we infer general laws from observation of specific events, and *deduction*, by which we explain specific events as resulting from general laws and initial conditions. The Aristotelian approach to knowledge resulted in the division of natural phenomena into categories, groups, or logical structures. This approach supported a *reductionist* approach in Western science – analyzing phenomena by dismantling them into smaller and smaller units. In contrast, Eastern cultures have been characterized by more *holistic* thinking – the idea that the whole cannot be fully understood simply through understanding its parts.

Western science was developed upon the premise that the universe is governed by fundamental laws that humans can discover by a process of reduction. For example, biologists seek to understand life processes by identifying the molecules that make up living organisms and understanding how these molecules behave; physicists seek to understand the nature of the universe by searching for subatomic particles and defining the forces by which these particles interact. Inherent in the reductionist approach to science has been the concept of *determinism* – the idea that given a particular set of initial conditions, the outcome of an event is predetermined by fundamental laws.

The experimental method of science (often called the "scientific method‘) rests upon these traditions. In this approach, scientists use deductive and inductive reasoning to infer the existence of general principles. Then, to test whether a principle is truly general, a scientist uses the principle as the premise of a testable hypothesis – an "if-then" statement whose truth can be tested experimentally. The scientist then designs an experiment in which most independent variables (factors that could affect the outcome) are either physically held constant (as in a laboratory) or statistically controlled (for example, by making sure that two random samples of survey respondents do not differ in some unintended way that might influence their responses). The scientist purposely alters one independent variable and analyzes the effect of this alteration on the outcome of the experiment (i.e., measurements of the dependent variable). Through repeated experiments, the scientist develops generalizable relationships between independent variables and the dependent variable.

As in other areas of science, biomedical and behavioral scientists studying addictions traditionally have taken a reductionist approach, focusing on the molecular basis of addictions in the individual. As a result, much of the scientific basis for prevention of alcohol-involved problems rests upon a reductionist and deterministic perspective on alcohol use and associated problems. The site of an alcohol problem is believed to be the individual drinker, who consumes alcohol in large quantities, sometimes in a compulsive and dependent fashion, as a result of specific factors that can be isolated and studied separately. Thus, alcohol problems are seen as being caused by "flawed" people – alcoholics, addicts, dependent persons, the poor, persons from broken families, incompletely socialized individuals, and psychologically damaged or genetically disadvantaged persons. Accordingly, the traditional goal of prevention has been to identify individuals who drink excessively or in a compulsive and dependent fashion, and to identify them early enough to prevent a natural progression to more and more destructive drinking.

In recent years, scientists in many fields have come to recognize the important role of chance in the course of natural phenomena. They have come to believe that rather than determining the outcomes of events, natural laws only describe the likelihoods (probabilities) of various possible outcomes. If the probability of one particular outcome is so high that scientists never happen to observe any other outcomes, the principle looks like an absolute law – the outcome appears to be predetermined. As scientists study increasingly complex systems, with many interacting components, the role of chance in affecting the outcome of each interaction becomes more and more important, and the overall behavior of the system becomes less and less predictable. In highly complex systems, such as social or ecological systems, scientists are finding that the principles arrived at through a reductionist approach do not in fact help them successfully predict the overall behavior of the system.

"Chaos" is a term used to express the complex dynamics of natural systems, be they in physics, chemistry, biology, ecology, economics, or social sciences. (For examples of the application of chaos theory in various fields, see Davies, 1989, on physics; Arthur, 1990, on economics; Perelson & Kauffman, 1990, on molecular biology; Nicolis & Prigogine, 1989, and Devaney, 1989, on the theory of complexity; and Axelrod, 1984, on social system adaptation. For a popular introduction to the concept of chaos, see Waldrup, 1992.) Chaotic and random behavior of complex systems is a natural feature of the world, not an exception to deterministic rules. Seemingly small changes in the conditions affecting a natural complex

system (such as social and economic systems) may result in major transformations in the system's structure and dynamics that could not have been
predicted through a reductionist approach. Complex natural systems are
by nature adaptive, transformational, and unpredictable.

This new paradigm has stimulated renewed interest in the study of
complex adaptive systems – systems that respond to external and internal
conditions and forces by evolving and transforming themselves over time.
(For discussion of the concept of the complex adaptive system, see Holland,
1975; Kauffman, 1991, 1993, 1995; Casti, 1992, 1994; and Stonier & Yu,
1994.) *Adaptation* refers to a system's inherent ability to accommodate to
changes or disturbances, arising from within the system or from the external
environment. Clearly, adaptation is a fundamental attribute of all living
organisms, as well as the social structures in which human beings live.

This book proposes an approach to prevention of alcohol-involved
problems from a systems dynamics perspective, in which the community is
studied and understood as a complex adaptive system. Several key terms
are useful in describing the community as a complex adaptive system.
Dynamic refers to the inherent nature of communities to change over time: a
dynamic system never stands still. *Complexity* means that multiple elements, levels, interactions, and subsystems are continually operating within the community. This complexity gives rise to the community's ability to
adapt. *Adaptation* refers to the transformational nature of communities –
their ability to adjust to both internal and external forces. The community is
continually adjusting to new conditions and input, and it is capable of
evolving into new and unpredictable structural arrangements. Because the
community is a complex adaptive system, mechanistic and deterministic
approaches to social and economic systems are inadequate to explain and
predict the occurrence of alcohol-involved problems in the community. At
worst, mechanistic and deterministic approaches are misleading and potentially destructive.

A new paradigm for prevention

A new paradigm for prevention of alcohol-involved problems is needed
now and for the 21st century. The following propositions are a useful
starting point:

- Alcohol (and other drug) problems are the natural result (output) of
  dynamic, complex, and adaptive systems called "communities."
- Working only with high-risk individuals or small groups produces, at
  best, short-term reductions in alcohol problems, because the system

will produce replacements for individuals who leave high-risk status, and the system will adapt to changes in the composition and behavior of subgroups and populations.

- Interventions in complex adaptive systems do not always yield the desired results, and they often produce undesired and unexpected outcomes that are counterintuitive ("not what we thought would happen").
- The most effective prevention strategies are those that seek to alter the system that produces alcohol problems.
- Prevention strategies historically have been "single solutions'; that is, they have attempted to accomplish a goal by one (usually massive) program or strategy, rather than by concurrent, mutually reinforcing approaches.
- Without an understanding of the community as a dynamic system – that is, without a model that increases our ability to understand and effectively change the system – it is unlikely that effective long-term prevention of alcohol problems will occur in practice.

Simply adding the word "community" to our prevention vocabulary is insufficient to accomplish the needed paradigm shift. In particular, scientists and practitioners in alcohol problem prevention must recognize that open, dynamic community systems adapt and adjust to their interventions, making lasting change difficult to achieve. Likewise, simply drawing boxes and arrows does not make a system. The community "system" is popularly illustrated by lines that connect "everything to everything." Such "system" drawings represent our ignorance and *naïveté*, not our appreciation and understanding.

Without an understanding of the dynamic, adaptive nature of the community system, one might develop explanations for the apparently stable oscillation of community alcohol consumption around a naturally occurring level. However, when consumption diverges from this level and establishes a new, different level, understanding is foiled. Over the short term, the natural oscillation appears to represent a stable, unchanging system. But either exogenous factors (from outside the system) or unpredictable (probabilistic) natural forces from within transform the system, and a new consumption level is established. It is the potential for such adaptive transformations that best characterizes community systems of alcohol use and alcohol problems.

Complex adaptive systems can never be fully understood by dismantling them into their basic components: the whole is greater than the sum of its parts. Scientific knowledge about alcohol use and alcohol problems, accumulated in piecemeal fashion, is fragmented. We understand alcohol problems and processes in isolation, but our knowledge of the larger picture is more limited. The community system is best understood as a whole composed of a set of interacting parts or subsystems. Each subsystem has its own organizing processes that influence, and in turn are influenced by, other subsystems. The entire system is organized at yet a higher level that transcends the organizing process of any one subsystem.

A systems perspective on alcohol-involved problems at the community level can assist researchers and help policy-makers at local and national levels, including legislative staff, elected officials, social and health workers, and prevention program specialists, to design effective local strategies for prevention of alcohol-involved problems. A national perspective cannot effectively guide interventions at the local level. To develop effective community-level prevention, policy-makers must understand how each of the community's subsystems influences alcohol use and thus contributes to alcohol-involved problems.

The catchment-area approach

Increasingly popular worldwide are community-based approaches to problem prevention that are best characterized as "catchment-area approaches." From the catchment-area perspective, a "community" is viewed as a set or sets of persons with adverse behaviors or associated risks with respect to the target problem, and the prevention effort is intended to reduce or eliminate these behaviors or risks. The model is straightforward: find the persons at risk (or identify the risk factors that individuals may possess), then educate, treat, or serve them to reduce the individual risk to each person so identified.

An example of a catchment approach might be prevention of cirrhosis mortality in a neighborhood with a transient, low-income population. The city or a local service organization would target this neighborhood and seek to reduce the drinking levels of identified chronic heavy drinkers by establishing a recovery center. In another example of a catchment-area approach, use of alcohol among students of a local middle school might be targeted and approached through strategies aimed at increasing the skills of pre-adolescents for resisting peer pressure to drink, developing alternative after-school activities, and implementing school-based and family-focused alcohol education programs. This approach ignores the role of retail sales of alcohol to young people, and its prevention activities generally do not affect community members not directly involved with these targeted populations.

The catchment-area approach employs strategies to alter individual decisions and behavior or to provide direct services to targeted individuals. The favored alcohol problem prevention efforts are education-based activities, with social and physical (and sometimes economic) reinforcement, and early identification of and intervention with individual heavy drinkers. Prevention efforts often include mass media announcements, focus groups, targeted communication, health promotion, health awareness campaigns, and physician education. Other potential components are one-on-one and group treatment, and counseling.

Most heart disease and cancer community prevention trials have employed a catchment-area approach of some form. The targets of these trials have been well-defined states or conditions with which individual residents of a community can be accurately associated. For example, if heavy smoking is the target, then heavy smokers can be identified, and education programs for smoking reduction and cessation can be directed at these individuals. Community heart disease prevention projects make effective use of the disease's links with diet, exercise, smoking, and genetics; they identify individuals who are at risk because of one or more of these factors and help them to adjust or moderate their behaviors to reduce the risk.

However, in the case of alcohol problem prevention, the catchment-area perspective has clear limitations. Although heavy dependent users (alcoholics) do have the greatest individual risk rates for most alcohol problems, they are not collectively the largest at-risk group. Their absolute numbers are so small that they contribute only modestly to most aggregate alcohol-related problems. Infrequent and moderate users of alcohol, who are not currently nor ever likely to be dependent on alcohol, account for a greater number of alcohol-involved traumas, such as traffic crashes, falls, or drownings (Edwards et al., 1994). In particular, young people account for a disproportionately large number of alcohol-involved traffic crashes and accidental injuries. Most addicted heavy drinkers continue this drinking pattern throughout their lives without ever experiencing an alcohol-involved traffic crash or encounter with the police. On the other hand, an 18–year-old with limited driving and drinking experience may cause a serious traffic crash with only a small amount of alcohol in the blood system. Physical and cognitive impairment begins as soon as the body begins to metabolize ethanol. Impairment increases as more ethanol enters the blood, and the individual can become increasingly impaired as drinking continues. The rate of impairment is a function of such factors as drinking experience and alcohol tolerance, body weight, rate of alcohol intake, and the amount of food consumed with the alcohol.

Most alcohol-involved problem events are stochastic; that is, they are probabilistic and time-dependent. The probability that any given drinker at any specific time will experience an alcohol-involved problem event usually is quite low. For example, an alcohol-impaired driver's chance of being stopped and arrested is estimated to be 1 in 2000 events on average. However, the chances of a traffic crash following drinking are quite high (Fell, 1983; Zobeck, 1986). *Alcohol-involved problems are not simply the results of actions of a set of definable high-risk individuals; rather, they are the accumulative result of the structure and interactions of complex social, cultural, and economic factors within the community system.*

The community system perspective

Alternatively, a "community" can be viewed as a set or sets of persons engaged in shared socio-cultural-politico-economic processes, which interact to such an extent that prevention efforts, to be effective, must be directed towards system-wide structures and processes. Because of its greater difficulty, the community system approach towards community problem prevention is less popular than the catchment-area approach. However, alcohol and other drug problems are the outcomes of processes driven and sustained by the community at large. These processes potentially affect all members of the community, but produce adverse effects in certain groups more than in others (because of individual and environmental factors that contribute to disproportionate exposure or increased susceptibility). From the community system perspective, the intention is to reduce the *collective risk* through appropriate interventions affecting community processes. As Churchman (1979) observed:

On the broadest level, the systems approach belongs to a whole class of approaches to managing and planning our human affairs with the intent that we as a living species conduct ourselves properly in this world. Everyone adopts at least one such approach during her/his life, even if he/she is a recluse, an agnostic, a nihilist.

Many public health and social problems are best addressed from a community system perspective. For example, there is little evidence that adolescents' decisions about criminal behavior and the pursuit of "criminal careers" are strictly the consequences of individual malfunctioning. Psychological, social, cultural, economic, and physical environmental factors can all contribute to producing the young criminal. To date, efforts to reduce youth crime rates through individual-focused counseling and education or through law enforcement and the courts have not proven successful. (For further discussion of prevention of adolescent criminality, see Whitehead & Lab, 1989.)

Aspects of systems strategies have been employed in community public health initiatives, including some heart disease and cancer prevention trials. For example, public health projects have succeeded in getting low-fat alternatives offered on restaurant menus, low-salt food products made available and prominently displayed in grocery stores, warning labels on the hazards of smoking installed at points of sale for cigarettes, and the number of non-smoking areas in public spaces and in the workplace increased. Some community health trials have employed public policy approaches that mandate the availability of low-fat food alternatives, increase the retail price of cigarettes, or legally restrict availability of cigarettes by banning cigarette machines.

With respect to alcohol problem prevention, the community system perspective differs from the catchment-area perspective in several important ways:

(1) Rather than addressing a single problem behavior or condition, it simultaneously considers a potentially wide-ranging set of alcohol-involved problems.
(2) Rather than focusing on individuals at risk, it studies the entire community in concert.
(3) Rather than basing prevention strategies on single assumptions about deterministic behavior, it employs interventions that alter the social, cultural, economic, and physical environment in such a way as to promote shifts away from conditions that favor the occurrence of alcohol-involved problems.

Understanding the community as a complex, adaptive system for the purpose of alcohol problem prevention

The community is a dynamic system. The complex adaptive community system is energized by people, as well as other sources of energy, including raw materials, money, information, and language. With respect to alcohol-involved problems, the system changes and adapts as new people enter the community system and others leave; as alcoholic beverage marketing and promotion evolve; and as social and economic conditions, such as employment and disposable income, change. The degree to which alcohol use is a part of routine life in the community will strongly influence the types and

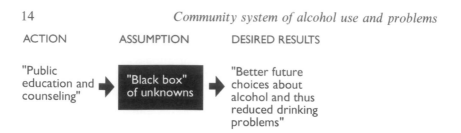

Figure 1.1 The traditional approach to alcohol problem prevention.

rates of alcohol problems the community system produces, given its current organizing structure.

Given the community system's ability to adapt to change, no single
prevention program, no matter how good, can sustain its impact, particularly if it does not result in system-level changes (see Wallack, 1981; Holder
& Wallack, 1986). Even if high-risk individuals (e.g., alcoholics) are identified and somehow "fixed," as long as the system structure remains unchanged, it will naturally generate replacements. The community system
approach has stimulated development of new prevention strategies to
modify community system structures, environments, and contexts from
which alcohol problems result.

Traditional approaches to alcohol problem prevention, whether as extreme as Prohibition or as contemporary as the use of television for public
education, have one thing in common: a basic (one might say simplistic)
belief that if a certain action is taken, a specific predictable result will
follow. Specifically, traditional approaches to alcohol problem prevention
are based on a set of assumptions about how people behave as individuals
or as groups. For example, one common proposition is that if people are
told about the dangers of drinking to excess, they will tend not to do so.
The traditional approach is illustrated in Fig. 1.1, where actions shown on
the left (e.g., public education and counseling) are assumed to have the
predictable and desired results on the right (e.g., better future choices about
alcohol and, thus, reduced drinking problems). In the middle, actions and
results are linked by a "black box" of unknown mechanisms. To the degree
that our guesses and assumptions about the workings of the "black box"
are correct, the desired results will occur. However, evaluation of community education prevention projects often shows that the prevention actions
have not yielded the desired results, and that many other factors outside
the control or concern of the project are at work. (For summaries of
research on this issue, see Blane, 1974; Moskowitz, 1989; and Holder, 1994.)

In a community system approach, drinking and its consequences are

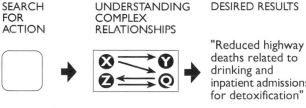

SEARCH FOR ACTION → UNDERSTANDING COMPLEX RELATIONSHIPS → DESIRED RESULTS "Reduced highway deaths related to drinking and inpatient admissions for detoxification"

Figure 1.2 Systems approach to alcohol prevention.

considered to be part of a system (a complex network). Ackoff & Emery (1972) gave us, over 20 years ago, a good definition of a system: "A set of interrelated elements, each of which is related directly or indirectly to every other element, and no subset of which is unrelated to any other subset." A community system approach requires some understanding of the black box. Our problem is how to develop an understanding or model that will organize what we know about the community system – its structure and dynamics. To usefully model the community system, we need not have all information about everything – we need only be aware of our information limitations. Figure 1.2 illustrates that the community is approached as a complex system which produces such problems as highway deaths or hospital admissions. An understanding of the community system then enables us to identify and test strategies that have the potential to reduce such problems.

The need for models of the community as a complex adaptive system

Without an integrating conceptual structure, information about the community remains a hodgepodge of fragments. Knowledge is a collection of observations, practices, and conflicting incidents. A model is an abstraction of reality that contains the most salient portions of the available knowledge – the variables of interest. Thus, a model of the community as a system is a structure (or theory) that can organize and synthesize the best available information relating to community dynamics with respect to the phenomenon of interest (in our case, alcohol-involved problems).

The general nature of complex systems (e.g., all social systems, such as urban areas, governments, corporations, international trade, and human service systems) involves a number of important and little-understood characteristics. Forrester (1969) defined a complex system as a "high-order, multiple-loop, nonlinear feedback structure." The *order* of a system refers to the number of levels (states or conditions) that are needed to describe it. For example, an urban area might be described with respect to such factors as income, revenue, population density, employment, health, welfare, poverty, social services, blight, construction, natural resources, energy, and social, physical, and economic stability. A system with a large number of levels is referred to as a complex or "high-order" system. *Multiple-loop* refers to the interaction of a large number of feedback loops within the system. *Feedback* refers to the flow of information (or other resources) from one level of the system to another and the effects of that flow on factors or decisions that control another level (element) of the system.

Positive feedback loops are growth-producing processes, by which growth generates further action that results in further growth. For example, population growth, and housing and highway construction can form a positive feedback loop, whereby population growth stimulates construction, which in turn stimulates additional population growth. Negative feedback loops tend to regulate the system towards some objective or to constrain tendencies to grow (or decline) without limit. The control of heating with a thermostat is an example of a negative loop: the thermostat compares the actual temperature to the desired (set) temperature and activates the furnace when the temperature drops below that level, to maintain a relatively constant (equilibrium) temperature. An example of negative feedback in an urban area is the use of zoning to attempt to limit housing development. In the community system, a number of positive and negative feedback loops are operating to influence alcohol use and alcohol problems, but the system has the potential to break out of existing "equilibrium" conditions and be transformed into a new arrangement.

Although planners and community leaders may intuitively appreciate that alcohol-involved problems result from many diverse factors, they generally do not have at their disposal the technology to translate intuitive understandings into concrete relationships. Thus, policy-makers must make decisions amidst considerable complexity, and they need tools to assist them in making the best use of available resources. Such tools would enable them to bring empirical and theoretical knowledge to bear on understanding the complex network of factors surrounding a set of alcohol problems, and estimating the likely impact of interventions in specific situations.

Decision-makers in the military and in industry recognized some time ago the benefit of computer modeling as a tool to aid in making decisions under uncertain conditions. *Computer modeling*, or *simulation*, involves constructing a mathematical model that represents reality and using the computer to manipulate the model in order to make projections of likely future consequences of events or actions. Computer models are causal approximations of the real world, based on and reflecting the best available data and experience. In other words, the computer model is designed to "act like" the real world, to enable us to predict the results of alternative courses of action (or inaction). Computer simulation can provide answers to the question, If I implement problem-prevention strategy X, what is most likely to happen? Furthermore, a model can be altered as new observations and findings become available. Computer modeling is a research and policy evaluation technique that has been used for at least three decades to investigate problems and changes in problem indicators as a result of system-level shifts in conditions. For further discussion of the principles and methods of systems dynamics, see Forrester, 1969, and Pugh, 1973. For a more general discussion of computer simulation, see Law & Kelton, 1982, Payne, 1982, and Hamilton et al., 1969.

Causal models can play an especially important role in the social sciences, where controlled experiments are not appropriate or possible. Their use in the study of social systems has been summarized by Ackoff & Emery (1972), who made the following observation:

In a sense the researcher into the operations of many social systems is in a situation similar to that of the early astronomers; the system they studied also seemed to be infinitely complex and yet incapable of being subjected to experimentation. However, astronomers eventually developed mathematical representations (models) of the systems, and analyzed or conducted experiments on these models. Today such experiments are called 'simulations.'

Because a computer model represents an explicit statement of theory, it can be used to test hypotheses. Even if a model has not been empirically validated, it still can be used to examine the implications of a theory. For example, if a researcher develops an explanatory theory of the relationship between the price of alcohol, changes in patterns of alcohol sales, and changes in alcohol use and social values about drinking, a model can be developed to explore this theory even if adequate data are not available to test it. If a model has been validated empirically, it can be used to test hypotheses about possible changes to reduce alcohol problems in the community system.

Although computer modeling has often been used in other areas of research, including business, economics, health care, retail sales, and defense, it has rarely been employed in the development of the science of alcohol problem prevention. Dynamic computer modeling is a technique for developing causal understanding of the complex community system of which alcohol use and abuse are a part. (For further discussion of the role of computer modeling in public policy about heroin, see Levin, Roberts &

Hirsch, 1975; and in alcohol problem prevention research see Summers & Harris, 1978; Holder & Blose, 1983, 1987, 1988.)

The mathematical structure of a computer model of the community system reflects the researcher's theory of how the community functions. When research observations and findings are expressed as a set of well-defined variables, and specific, well-defined relationships among variables, they can be incorporated into a computer model, which can then be used as a tool to interrelate and interpret the observations and findings. In brief, the model can be composed of a series of causal relationships derived from a variety of sources:

(1) Published scientific literature (the preferred source).
(2) Statistical analyses of data, specifically to examine variables and relationships for the model that have not been explored in the scientific literature.
(3) Expert judgment and theory.

As with classical experimentation, testing through computer simulation involves introducing specific changes or "treatments" into the model system, observing the outcome, and using statistical tests to determine whether any differences observed are significantly different from past observations, or from a control group or situation (i.e., the differences are not due to random error). To test a given prevention strategy in a community system model, the researcher identifies specific system variables that are to be altered (by the proposed prevention strategy) and conducts a computer simulation in which a validated model "acts like" the actual community system over a specified period of time. Through the simulation, the model produces information about the changes in system behavior associated with the alterations in system variables made by the researcher.

Computer modeling of a dynamic system is a uniquely powerful tool for understanding the underlying mechanisms of community processes and predicting change. It allows researchers to answer questions that cannot be addressed directly via other statistical techniques commonly used in the social sciences.

In the field of substance abuse, statistical techniques traditionally are used to determine static empirical relationships between variables. For example, cross-sectional data analysis techniques may be used to derive findings from a school survey or a community survey. The results of such an analysis are, of course, applicable only to the population that was sampled. Even if a nationally representative survey is conducted, the results are generalizable only to the time at which the survey was made. For example, survey results cannot tell us anything about the situation ten years prior to the survey, nor can they predict the situation ten years in the future.

Time-series or longitudinal statistical techniques provide information about changes over time in the variables under study. Standard time-series and spatial analysis following Box & Jenkins (1976), Tiao & Box (1981) and McCleary et al. (1980) establish the empirical patterns and cycles in time-series data. Such techniques have been used successfully in alcohol policy analyses (Wagenaar, 1986; Blose & Holder, 1987; and Wagenaar & Holder, 1991, 1995). However, they primarily establish historical patterns and cycles of the time series itself; they do not identify the underlying causal relationships that produced the series.

Although conventional multivariate statistical techniques might be used to derive parameter values used in dynamic system models, the models bear little resemblance to these statistical techniques. The systems dynamics approach does not involve curve fitting; rather, it requires first the conceptual specification and then the mathematical specification of a dynamic system in which variables interact with one another over time in an iterative fashion.

Simulation models can contribute to alcohol problem prevention research in at least four areas:

(1) *Enhancing understanding of the community as a system.* Numerous studies have analyzed various aspects of alcohol-related problems, but seldom have efforts been made to integrate these findings. At the same time prevention programs and activities (no matter how well planned or managed) are operating, other uncontrolled factors, such as social custom or changes in economic factors, can obscure or impede the programs' potential impact. Because a complex system behaves in unexpected ways, efforts to prevent or reduce alcohol problems can have results that are unintended and possibly undesired. Development of an integrating structure or model that increases our understanding of the system as a whole will enhance our ability to design effective prevention programs.
(2) *Identifying the implications of existing information, as well as gaps in our knowledge.* By enabling us to interrelate research findings and explore their implications, a model will increase our understanding of

specific alcohol problems and their prevention, as well as helping us to identify the limits of our knowledge and, thus, our research needs.

(3) *Expanding available analytical tools.* Most statistical techniques used in social, behavioral, and biomedical research cannot adequately account for the dynamic interaction of system variables. When variables are studied in isolation, it is difficult to explore the precise linkages between actions and effects, to anticipate unexpected results, or to assess the impacts of concurrently operating prevention efforts. Forrester (1969) cautioned that the time correlation between variables in complex systems can lead one to infer cause-and-effect relationships in cases where variables may be simply moving together as a consequence of dynamic interactions in the system.

(4) *Allowing new research findings to be incorporated.* A system model can be updated to incorporate new knowledge as it becomes available.

Computer models of systems can be used to investigate the interplay of system variables and relationships identified by research to be potentially important. Thus, one can use such models to investigate complex linkages between cause and effect, to anticipate results that might otherwise be unexpected, and to more fully assess the effects of two or more prevention programs operating simultaneously. Researchers can use these models to construct subsystems that reflect alternate theories or explanations for important processes.

The utility of community system models and one example

Researchers can use community system models to explore structural relationships that reflect alternative theories or explanations of important processes (e.g., the relationship between the availability of alcohol and its consumption by one or more groups within the community). Policymakers can use such models to explore the potential impacts of alternative intervention strategies before finalizing their prevention plans.

The interests of researchers and prevention policy-makers are similar, but not identical. Policy-makers are interested not merely in understanding the general effects of a particular strategy in the past, but in anticipating its future impact in a specific situation. Conventional research and evaluation studies do not provide the *prospective* information that policy-making requires. Traditional research methods often are best suited for examining only a small number of variables in isolation from other factors.

Studying specific alcohol uses and alcohol-involved problems in isolation provides little reliable basis for predicting the effects of specific future prevention interventions.

Effective public policy to reduce alcohol-involved problems is best formulated when decision-makers are aware of the range of existing prevention alternatives and their potential effects. However, policy often cannot await the completion of definitive research analyses. Further, given the nature of scientific research, it is unlikely that sufficient data will ever exist to permit prevention strategies to be selected with complete certainty of their outcome. Community prevention planners wish to make use of the best available scientific research, but the results of most prevention research are published in technical journals and reports in a form that makes their practical application difficult. Even if prevention planners had the time and resources to review such research, they would still have the problem of how to make use of the information in their planning. That is, they would still not know the likely results of applying specific prevention strategies in their community or geographic area. Thus, a community prevention planner requires knowledge of the viable alternatives for reducing alcohol problems, and a means of forecasting the long-term results that might occur in a given community if any one or a mix of these alternatives were implemented. One example of a computer-based systems-dynamics model of the community is *SimCom* (Simulated Community), which has been developed and field tested by the Prevention Research Center, Berkeley, California, for the past 15 years. *SimCom* is described in Chapter 8. Many types of complex adaptive system models could be developed to assist alcohol problem prevention research and practice. This book does not describe *SimCom* in detail, as the specifics of this model, and its structure and application are not central to this book's purpose, which is to describe the rationale for complex adaptive system approaches and their utility. Nonetheless, this book uses the community structures on which *SimCom* is based to provide a perspective and a conceptual model for a systems approach to community alcohol problem prevention.

The community system and its subsystems

The community system (as used by *SimCom*) can be divided into interacting subsystems, which are natural groupings of factors and variables that research has shown to be important to an understanding of alcohol use and alcohol problems. Consumption is the central subsystem; it both affects and is affected by the other subsystems. To design effective prevention of

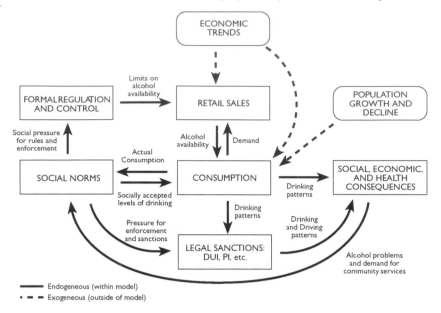

Figure 1.3 Conceptual model of alcohol use and alcohol problems.

alcohol problems, we must consider the interactions among these subsystems. Below, each subsystem is introduced, along with a brief description of how the subsystems interact. The following chapters of this book discuss each subsystem in turn. Figure 1.3 illustrates the complete community system, including typical interaction among the six subsystems.

Consumption Subsystem: alcohol use as a part of routine community life

This is the key subsystem of the community system. Patterns or distributions of alcohol consumption shift over time, and the differential effects of age and gender on consumption must be taken into account. The consumption distributions for each age and gender group can be divided into subgroups according to average daily consumption and the distribution of drinks consumed per drinking occasion. The consumption distributions for each age and gender group are affected by such factors as personal income, alcohol price, availability of alcohol, social acceptability or norms about consumption, and alcohol regulations, such as the legal age for drinking. Changes in these factors can produce corresponding changes in consumption (Brenner, 1975; Skog, 1986). When these factors change, the net effect of the changes determines a new value for average daily consumption, resulting in a shift in the consumption pattern for each age and gender group and the community as a whole.

Retail Sales Subsystem: alcohol availability and promotion

Alcohol as a commercial product is made available to consumers via retail sales outlets. These may be publicly licensed retail outlets (such as stores, pubs, or restaurants) or informal outlets (such as private homes, unlicensed establishments, or even roadside vendors, such as "moonshiners" or families producing and selling *pulque*). Depending on the alcohol beverage control laws, retail establishments may obtain licenses for the sale of alcohol for consumption at the location of the establishment (e.g., bars, pubs, restaurants, or arenas) or for the sale of alcohol in containers for consumption elsewhere (e.g., wine shops, liquor stores, supermarkets, or convenience stores) (Godfrey, 1988; Gruenewald, Ponicki & Holder, 1993). The number and types of outlets that are licensed to sell alcoholic beverages in a community are affected by population size and trends, prior per capita alcohol consumption in the community, and economic factors (e.g., average disposable income).

Formal Regulation and Control Subsystem: rules, administration, and enforcement

In most cultures, alcohol is regulated in one fashion or another. This subsystem reflects government rules and controls to regulate retail sales of alcohol. For example, restrictions might be placed on the number of new licenses of a given type, or on the days and hours of permitted retail sales, as a means of curbing availability of alcohol. Local communities also may regulate the densities of alcohol sales establishments through zoning (Wittman & Hilton 1987). The strengths of rules and regulations are affected by enforcement activities, and the severity of penalties for violations.

Social Norms Subsystem: community values and social influences that affect drinking

The Social Norms Subsystem reflects community values about alcohol. Social norms influence levels of alcohol consumption through both positive and negative feedback. "Positive feedback" describes the phenomenon whereby increases in consumption of alcohol over time are associated with increased acceptance of alcohol use. "Negative feedback" describes the phenomenon whereby increased consumption results in increased alcohol-involved problems and, consequently, in decreased social acceptance (Haskins, 1985; Partanen & Montonen, 1988). The influences of gender, ethnicity, and other sociocultural factors result in differing norms among subgroups within the community (Caetano, 1988; Corbett, Mora & Ames, 1991).

Legal Sanctions Subsystem: prohibited uses of alcohol

The Legal Sanctions Subsystem is organized to enforce rules against use of alcohol in specific contexts and situations. These may include (but not be limited to) drinking and driving, public intoxication and possession of alcohol, underage drinking, or drinking at specific sites (e.g., in public parks, on boats, on the beach, or in public facilities such as auditoriums and stadiums). In developed countries, a major aspect of this subsystem is enforcement of laws against drinking and driving (i.e., detection and punishment of persons who drive after or while drinking, as well as deterrence of this behavior). The distribution of driving events (i.e., vehicle trips) as a function of blood alcohol concentration (BAC) is influenced by community alcohol consumption, social norms, and the intensity and severity of enforcement of laws against drinking and driving (Ross, 1982; Homel, 1988). This distribution of driving events by blood alcohol concentration determines the frequency of alcohol-involved traffic problems, including driver fatalities and crashes resulting in injury.

Social, Economic, and Health Consequences Subsystem: community identification of and organized responses to alcohol problems

The consequences of drinking (e.g., numbers of alcohol-involved injuries or deaths, alcohol-involved workplace accidents, or cirrhosis deaths) are addressed in the Social, Economic, and Health Consequences Subsystem. Alcohol-involved mortality and morbidity reflect the health and injury risks associated with drinking. Risks of alcohol-involved problems vary by age, gender, and consumption group (Joksch, 1985; Roman, 1990; Anderson et al. 1993; and Anderson, 1995). Group-specific risk rates linked to levels of alcohol consumption determine the frequency of alcohol-associated deaths, illnesses, and injuries (Howland & Hingson, 1987, 1988; Cherpitel 1989, 1993). Increases in alcohol-involved mortality and morbidity can trigger social activity and, consequently, formal regulatory activity aimed at reducing consumption or behaviors associated with alcohol-involved problems. This subsystem also responds to the demand for social and health services related to drinking, and permits a community to track increases (or decreases) in provision of health and social services related to drinking. This aspect of the subsystem is concerned with such information as number of patients, treatment facilities and costs, waiting-list sizes, and average time in treatment.

Subsystem interactions

By reviewing the characteristics and internal dynamics of each of these subsystems, we develop a perspective of the community system. However, discussion of the subsystems individually does not reflect their interconnectedness, or "systemness." Here, we briefly summarize how these subsystems may interact.

The Consumption Subsystem both stimulates (provides input to) and receives input from other subsystems. The consumption of alcohol creates demand for alcohol as a retail product and thus stimulates the Retail Sales Subsystem. In turn, the Retail Sales Subsystem creates the opportunity for marketing and purchase of alcohol, thus stimulating consumption. Patterns of drinking influence patterns of drinking and driving, thus providing input to the Legal Sanctions Subsystem. Injuries and death caused by drinking and driving, together with other alcohol-involved chronic and acute health and safety problems in the community, provide input to the Social, Economic, and Health Consequences Subsystem, such as demand for emergency and inpatient hospital treatment and health services.

The Social Norms Subsystem establishes the community's values or norms about drinking and influences the patterns of drinking in the community. In turn, the current actual level of drinking sets a standard for the future acceptable level of drinking; that is, feedback exists between actual and acceptable levels of drinking. The Social Norms Subsystem reflects the concerns of the community about alcohol problems. For example, an increase in drinking and driving problems (themselves the result of patterns of drinking and driving influenced by the Social Norms Subsystem) can result in increased community concern. Increased community concern about drinking and driving (or at least the attention of a specific interest group, such as Mothers Against Drunk Driving) can, in turn, produce pressure (input to the Legal Sanctions Subsystem) to increase police surveillance and attention to enforcement of the laws against driving under the influence of alcohol (DUI), or to increase the frequency of DUI convictions and the severity of punishment in the court system. Similarly, community concerns about underage drinking can put pressure on the Formal Regulation and Control Subsystem for increased enforcement of laws against sales to underage persons.

The Formal Regulation and Control Subsystem reflects the community's desires about the type and level of formal controls over alcohol sales. This subsystem can define whether alcohol is legal or illegal (e.g., in Moslem societies, it is prohibited, whereas in France or Italy, it is a desired and valued aspect of routine living). Most industrialized countries establish rules and regulations concerning the types and forms of alcohol production and retail sales. Thus, depending upon social values, the forms of alcohol outlets can be controlled or restricted (e.g., via public monopolies on alcohol sales or restriction of the days and hours when retail sales are allowed). The Formal Regulation and Control Subsystem regulates the Retail Sales Subsystem, thus determining the overall level of alcohol availability (both formally and informally).

The Retail Sales Subsystem influences consumption by establishing the level of alcohol availability (as an input to the Consumption Subsystem). It also affects demand through sales promotion, setting of prices, and control over the convenience of alcohol's availability. The form and extent of the Retail Sales Subsystem is shaped (in some instances, dominated) by the regulations established in the Formal Regulation and Control Subsystem.

Alcohol-involved problems result from patterns of drinking, which are expressed in the Consumption Subsystem, and they occur in the Social, Economic, and Health Consequences Subsystem. Such problems are responded to by the community's existing social and health institutions. For example, alcoholics or alcohol-dependent persons create demand for alcohol recovery services, and alcohol-involved injuries create demand for emergency and trauma care.

In these ways, linkages are established among the six subsystems, as illustrated in Fig. 1.3. Although this simple description does not fully explore the nuances of the interrelationships among community subsystems, it does illustrate how relationships among subsystems are established. The status and nature of a subsystem at any point in time is influenced by the other subsystems with which it interacts; but at the same time, this subsystem can influence the status and nature of the other subsystems. In this fashion, a series of mutually influencing relationships (feedback loops) are established and maintained.

Overview and thesis of the book

The major thesis of this book is that the community is the "new frontier" for alcohol problem prevention and alcohol policy. In most developed countries, efforts to reduce alcohol problems have relied greatly on implementation of alcohol policies at the national level. Over the past 20 years, alcohol programs and policies have largely been directed at prevention at the national level via strategies of reduced alcohol availability. However, the development of the European Union, the General Agreement on Tariffs and Trade (GATT) treaty, and other international trade agreements have substantially weakened the potential for prevention via such national policies. In some cases, public monopolies on production and distribution of alcohol have been or will be eliminated. The spread of free-market economies and international trade agreements increases the need for prevention strategies at the local level.

In North America, with the independence of Canadian provinces and the individual US states, there is no national alcohol problem prevention policy. However in the US and Canada, considerable emphasis is placed on alcohol-problem prevention efforts at the local level. For example, in the US alone, over 500 communities have received demonstration grants in substance abuse prevention from the federal and state governments, and private foundations. The opportunity and need for prevention organized at the local or community level have never been greater.

Effective community-level alcohol policy strategies will often be quite different from the national policies, and their development will require a different point of view or perspective. Most prevention efforts organized at the local level fail to recognize the dynamic systems in which alcohol use and alcohol-involved problems exist. Thus, most current prevention programs either fail or produce only short-term effects.

This book will assist in establishing a new community systems paradigm that represents a clear break with individualistic and deterministic prevention perspectives. It seeks to provide a conceptual model of the overall community system and to assist those interested and responsible for alcohol problem prevention to recognize:

(1) The total system.
(2) Those forces that affect prevention but cannot be influenced by prevention strategies.
(3) Those factors that can be influenced in order to reduce problems.

Chapters 2 to 7 describe the six major subsystems of the community system, and explain how each subsystem influences alcohol use and alcohol-involved problems as it interacts with other subsystems. The book concludes with a discussion of how prevention planners can use a complex adaptive systems perspective to reduce alcohol problems in the community. The final chapter also demonstrates how the computer-based simulation model *SimCom* can be loaded to represent a real community and used to explore alternative strategies for alcohol problem prevention.

2

Consumption Subsystem

Introduction

Alcohol is consumed in most of the world's industrial cultures and in many non- or pre-industrial cultures. Some cultures have formal bans on alcohol, but in many, consumption of alcohol is a part of routine community life. Although the proportion of people who elect to abstain from alcohol varies across communities and cultures, alcohol is likely to be consumed in some form by a significant percentage of the population where it is not forbidden. In a community system, drinking is manifested in the Consumption Subsystem.

Each member of a community can be described according to his or her patterns of drinking (including abstention), characterized by quantity and frequency of alcohol consumption and by rates of intoxication. Across the community as a whole, these individual drinking (or abstinence) patterns in the aggregate form consumption categories or distributions, which make up the Consumption Subsystem. Alcohol use within the community differs by age, gender, marital status, religious preference, and racial or ethnic heritage. Men usually consume more alcohol on average than do women. Youths, young adults, adults, and the elderly exhibit distinct patterns of alcohol use. People from religious groups that prohibit alcohol use (e.g., Muslims, Mormons, or Southern Baptists in the US) consume less alcohol than do people from religious groups with no such proscriptions. Within the US, whites, African-Americans, and Latinos differ in their drinking patterns.

The Consumption Subsystem is dynamic. Over time, people move from one consumption category to another, changing both frequency and quantity of alcohol consumption. For example, people alter their drinking patterns as a result of aging or changes in personal disposable income. Nonetheless, consumption categories within the subsystem may be self-perpetuating; for example, new drinkers may replace former drinkers who have begun to abstain.

The Consumption Subsystem is influenced by economic factors and the availability of alcohol. For example, consumption is influenced by the retail price of each type of alcoholic beverage (beer, wine, and distilled spirits) and by the numbers and types of outlets that sell alcohol for on-premises consumption (such as bars, pubs, or restaurants) or off-premises consumption (such as liquor or grocery stores). Consumption is the source of demand for alcohol in the Retail Sales Subsystem. In turn, the demand for alcohol is affected by retail sales practices, as described in Chapter 3.

The Consumption Subsystem also is influenced by the community's social values or norms related to drinking, including the levels of consumption considered socially acceptable. In general, where drinking is more acceptable, it is more widespread, and average consumption is higher. In turn, the prevailing level of alcohol consumption in the community reinforces the norms for acceptable levels of drinking. Thus, the Consumption Subsystem both influences and is influenced by the Social Norms Subsystem.

Drinking as a part of routine activity

Alcohol is a part of routine life in any community, even if the community formally prohibits the use and sale of alcohol. The role of drinking in the life of members of a given community is defined by the extent to which alcohol is available both socially and for retail sale, and is consumed by members of the community. The availability of alcohol, both through retail outlets and in social contexts, influences the overall level of alcohol consumption; in turn, the level of consumption influences the availability of alcohol. The more alcohol is accepted as a part of routine community life – an integral part of the community's social and economic activities – the more it forms part of natural social interactions in the life of the average community member, and the more likely any community member is to drink.

Alcohol's role in routine community life, and the relationship between its availability and consumption, are illustrated by changes in per capita consumption of alcohol around the world. See Simpura (1995) for a discussion of changes in alcohol consumption across the world. For example, in the US over the past 10 to 15 years, drinking in public places, especially restaurants, has increased. This change in consumption is likely to be due to an increase in the frequency with which people go out of the house to participate in leisure activities, especially at night. In this example, drinking patterns have been influenced both by changes in routine personal activities (e.g., people increasingly going out to eat) and by the convenient availability of alcohol in public settings. (For further discussion, see Gruenewald, Ponicki & Holder, 1993; Gruenewald et al., 1995.)

Within the realms of routine activity, drinking choices (location, beverage, and quantity to consume) depend on many factors. For example, the desire to drink while eating at a restaurant is influenced by the availability of alcohol at the restaurant (e.g., only beer may be available) and the prices of beverages at that restaurant. The desire to consume alcohol is also influenced by income and relative costs; for example, an individual may choose to drink at home rather than in a restaurant in order to save money or to be able to drink more alcohol per unit cost.

The role of alcohol in routine activities also can be related to the risk of alcohol-involved problems. Parker (1995) and Parker & Rebhun (1995) showed that as drinking becomes a part of routine activities away from home, the risk of victimization can increase. Casswell, Fang Zhang & Wyllie (1993) found that in New Zealand the number of self-reported alcohol-involved problems varies according to the choice of drinking location (hotel, pub, or club) and the amount of alcohol typically consumed. Stockwell, Lange & Rydon (1993) found that in Australia fights and arguments among male heavy drinkers are more likely to occur at bars and pubs than elsewhere. Parker (1995) predicted that alcohol consumption patterns directly affect homicide rates. See, in addition, Lenke (1990) concerning alcohol and violence in the Nordic Countries and France.

Consumption classifications

Within a community's population of drinkers (say, anyone who consumes at least one drink per year), the pattern of alcohol consumption varies from one person to the next. For example, an individual may drink small amounts each day, large amounts only at the weekend, small amounts only occasionally, or large amounts daily. Such a pattern, which takes into account both the quantity consumed and the frequency at which it is consumed, has been called the "quantity frequency of consumption" (Cahalan, Cisin & Crossley, 1969; Cahalan & Room, 1974). By defining a set of quantity frequency categories and assigning individual consumption patterns to these categories, one can describe the community's overall consumption pattern. For example, Cahalan & Cisin (1968) developed five

Table 2.1. *Three consumption classifications*

| Alternative | Mean daily consumption of absolute ethanol (oz.) [Milliliters of absolute ethanol] (Expected percentage of the US population) | | | |
	Class 1	Class 2	Class 3	Class 4
1	0.000 [0.000] (30–35)	0.100–0.219 [2.957–6.477] (30–35)	0.220–0.999 [6.506–29.544] (25)	1.000+ [29.574+] (10)
2	0.000–0.219 [0.000–6.477] (60–70)	0.220–0.999 [6.506–29.544] (25)	1.000–1.999 [29.574–59.118] (6)	2.000+ [59.148+] (4)
3	0.000–0.219 [0.000–6.477] (60–70)	0.220–0.499 [6.506–14.757] (10–15)	0.500–1.999 [14.787–59.118] (15–20)	2.000+ [59.148+] (4)

consumption classes based on the following five categories of consumption quantity and frequency:

- "Heavy drinkers" – those who drink large quantities at least two to three times per month or small quantities at least three times per day. "Moderate drinkers" – those who drink large quantities about once per month or small quantities about twice per day. "Light drinkers" – those who drink medium quantities about once per month or small quantities once per day. "Infrequent drinkers" – those who drink any quantity less than once per month, but at least once per year. "Abstainers" – those who drink any quantity less than once per year or who never drink.

Other classifications can be (and have been) developed; how the quantity frequency categories are defined depends on how the classification will be used.

Alternatively, if consumption is measured in terms of absolute ethanol consumed per unit time (e.g., daily), the alcohol consumption of a population will form a continuous distribution (as discussed in more detail below). This continuous distribution can be arbitrarily divided into consumption categories. Table 2.1 shows three alternative consumption classifications based on average ounces (oz.) of absolute ethanol consumed daily with the milliliter (ml) equivalent in brackets, i.e., 1 oz. equals 29.574 ml. As described in Miller, Heather & Hall (1991), there are a number of national conventions for describing a "standard drink" in terms of absolute alcohol. As pointed out for the US, a typical drink is usually 0.500 US oz. or 14.787 ml (by volume). This book will use "drink" to refer to 0.500 US oz. of absolute alcohol, that is 14.787 ml or 11.671 grams (g) (by weight).

Alternative 1

This classification was used in the US national alcohol consumption surveys from 1964 to 1976. The purpose of consumption surveys is to describe the general population's drinking patterns. Because the majority of the US population are light drinkers, this classification gives a good picture of the distribution of consumption by distinguishing between categories of lighter drinkers, while lumping together moderate and heavy drinkers.

Alternative 2

This classification distinguishes between degrees of heavy drinking by providing separate categories for heavy (class 3) and very heavy (class 4) drinkers. Most individuals labeled "alcoholic" would be expected to fall into class 4. This classification allows comparison of two groups of high-risk drinkers. However, because approximately 90% of the US population falls into classes 1 and 2 (Johnson et al., 1977; Clark & Hilton, 1991), this classification provides little differentiation of consumption habits and associated risk for a large proportion of the population.

Alternative 3

Like alternative 2, this classification lumps abstainers and lighter drinkers into one category. Class 2 consists of what are often considered light to moderate drinkers, approximately 10 to 15% of the US population. Classes 3 and 4 consist of what are often considered heavy and very heavy drinkers. Thus, this classification distinguishes between groups of particular interest in terms of prevention. The *SimCom* model classifies consumption according to the four categories of alternative 3. These categories, based on ounces of absolute ethanol consumed per day, correspond to the following consumption levels: class 1 – less than three drinks per week; class 2 – at least three but fewer than seven drinks per week; class 3 – at least one but fewer than four drinks per day; and class 4 – four or more drinks per day.

Demographic and sociocultural differences in consumption patterns

Alcohol consumption surveys in most countries (see cross national survey results in Fillmore et al., 1991) have shown that age and gender groups have distinctive consumption patterns and that consumption varies by gender within an age group. Community drinking patterns can thus be described in terms of the distinctive drinking patterns of each age and gender group. As the age and gender mix of the community changes (e.g., the proportion of older or younger people in the community changes as a result of migration, births, or deaths), the overall community pattern (and level) of drinking can change.

Cahalan & Cisin (1968) and Cahalan & Room (1972) found clear empirical evidence of differences in US drinking patterns by age and gender groups, as well as by education, income, religion, and geographical region. Such findings have come from analysis of national drinking data and from community studies, such as those in Oakland, California (Knupfer & Room, 1964), San Francisco, California (Room, 1972), and Boston, Massachusetts (Wechsler, Demone & Gottlieb, 1978). More recent US studies have provided evidence of ethnic and minority differences from national consumption patterns (Clark & Midanik, 1982; Caetano & Medina-Mora, 1988; Clark & Hilton, 1991; Herd, 1991; Caetano, 1995).

Using data from two drinking panels in the US, Fillmore (1987*a*, *b*) reached these conclusions:

(1) The frequency of drinking at least once per year decreases with age.
(2) Decreases with age occur in the frequency and incidence of drinking at least once per week, and having three or more drinks at least occasionally.
(3) The frequency of drinking nearly every day is about the same across age groups, but the frequency of heavy drinking increases after 40, while its incidence decreases.
(4) The frequency of having five or more drinks at least once per week decreases with age.
(5) Decreases with age occur in the frequency and incidence of becoming intoxicated at least once per year, self-reported alcohol problems, and social complications associated with drinking.

Treno, Parker & Holder (1993) examined the relationship between changes in the age structure of the US and subsequent changes in per capita ethanol consumption from 1950 to 1987. Controlling for income, the divorce-tomarriage ratio, and the percent of women employed (as a surrogate for women's increased participation in the work force), they observed a statistically significant relationship using multivariate time-series analysis between the ratio of young to older males and per capita alcohol consumption among men.

Fillmore (1988) reviewed the past 70 years of cross-national longitudinal research on alcohol use throughout the life course. Using 41 longitudinal data sets on the general population from 15 countries, Fillmore et al. (1991) compared drinking patterns and problems within age and gender groups throughout the life course for persons representing different birth cohorts, historical epochs, and cultures. Both studies found the following patterns:

(1) Among males, alcohol consumption per occasion decreases with increasing age.
(2) Consumption level shows a strong "maturational effect," decreasing over time among men at younger ages in Canada, the UK, and the US; at middle ages in the Federal Republic of Germany; and at older ages in the US.
(3) In the US and Canada, consumption is likely to decrease among men in their early twenties.
(4) Mean consumption typically is lower among women than among men throughout the life course; men's per-occasion consumption is highest in the late teens and early twenties.
(5) Among US women, the stability of consumption per typical drinking occasion increases with age; the older the woman, the more likely her consumption during a typical occasion will remain the same over intervals ranging from 1 to 21 years.

These data on age- and gender-related drinking patterns and their stability across cultures provide additional evidence for the stability of the maturational effect: typically, as a person gets older, his or her drinking level reaches a peak and then declines. On average, women drink less than do men, and their drinking peaks later in life.

Age groups used in *SimCom*

Age is an important predictor of particular kinds of alcohol consumption and alcohol-involved problems, such as alcohol-involved accidental injuries and death among the young, and alcohol-related chronic disease in older drinkers. Seven age groups have been defined for use in *SimCom*.

(Alternative age groupings are, of course, possible.) The rationale for use of these seven age groups is as follows:

Age 13 to 17. Pre-adolescents and adolescents are grouped together to simplify the model. Generally, 13– to 15–year-olds do not drive, whereas some 16– and 17–year-olds are new drivers with substantially higher risks of traffic accidents. However, the 13–to–17 age group is characterized by dramatic increases in drinking frequency with age.

Age 18 to 20. This population is most affected by the minimum drinking age and often is characterized by heavy drinking per occasion.

Age 21 to 25. This population, along with the 18–to-20 age group, is characterized by high consumption levels, and high risk for accidental injuries and death associated with drinking (e.g., in drinking and driving crashes).

Age 26 to 34. This population characteristically shows the first marked drop in the rate and frequency of consumption and stabilization of life patterns of consumption. Heavier drinking begins to decline, and the percentage of abstainers increases.

Age 35 to 49. This population characteristically creates the heaviest demand for inpatient and outpatient care associated with heavy dependent drinking. Early death associated with patterns of heavy drinking first occurs in this age group.

Age 50 to 64. This population is characterized by an increasing trend toward abstention, and a large proportion of treated alcoholics and individuals who show the effects of long-term alcohol abuse.

Age 65 and over. Typically, the retired population experiences increased loneliness and isolation, and thus is at potential risk for heavy drinking. In general, this group is characterized by abstention; heavy drinking is likely to be a problem only in small subgroups. Alcohol-related deaths from chronic, degenerative disease are most likely to occur in this age group.

Cohort effects

All other things being equal, one might expect drinking patterns to be determined by age – or, more precisely, by life-cycle changes associated with various ages. One could hypothesize that as individuals get older, their drinking practices change in reasonably predictable ways, and that practices for a given age group are relatively stable over time (e.g., 18– to 20–year-olds in 1970 and 18– to 20–year-olds in 1980 would show similar drinking patterns). International collaborative drinking studies (e.g., Fillmore 1987*a*) have in fact shown consistent cross-cultural age-specific drinking patterns, apparently influenced by physical maturation and changes in metabolism, as well as by the cultural cues for each age group. However, similar age groups across years may also show differences in their drinking patterns, or "cohort effects."

A "cohort effect" for alcohol consumption is a pattern of drinking characteristic of the members of a particular age group which persists among that group of people as they move together into older age groups. At any time, age-specific drinking patterns may be modified by contemporaneous environmental factors, including economic conditions, cultural influences, and the accessibility of alcohol (e.g., the minimum age to purchase it). Broader social processes (such as increased education) or significant historical events (such as wars) also can significantly alter drinking patterns. The effects of such factors are probably greatest during the formative years of adolescence or young adulthood. Some of the drinking patterns of these age groups may be carried forward into adulthood. Thus, a cohort's initial drinking behavior and values, shaped by cultural and economic factors specific to the times, may influence the cohort's subsequent drinking patterns in ways independent of age. For example, people who were 20 to 25 years old in the 1940s, during World War II, may at that time have formed responses to alcohol and patterns of drinking quite different from those formed by 20- to 25-year-olds in the 1980s. These responses and drinking patterns may have continued to affect their consumption as they have moved into older age groups. As a cohort ages, cohort effects on drinking patterns continue to be mediated and modified by new, contemporaneous influences.

Glynn et al. (1985), using the panel data from the Normative Aging Study in the US, found evidence of a cohort effect on drinking patterns, separate from the effect of age. On the other hand, Fillmore (1987*a*) concluded that cohort membership did not affect age-specific drinking patterns of men in the mid to late 20th century in the US. In a more recent report, based upon cross-national longitudinal research, Fillmore et al. (1991) argued for historical, cultural, and cohort effects as explanations for cross-cultural variations in drinking. For example, Fillmore and her colleagues postulated that the more permissive the culture in which young men reach their peak alcohol consumption, the more stable their consumption will be over time.

Abstention

Non-drinkers make up an important part of any culture. About one-third of the US population abstain from alcohol, a proportion that has remained relatively stable during the past 60 years. This consumption pattern is unusual, both because this proportion of abstainers is significantly larger than in any other Western country and because it has remained stable during a period of increasing alcohol consumption (Room, 1983; Hilton, 1986; Hilton & Clark, 1991). Consumption of alcohol in the US increased annually from the end of World War II to the early 1980s, but has since declined (Clark & Hilton, 1991).

In the US, abstainers include relatively more women than men, relatively more older than younger people, relatively more low-income than higher-income individuals, and relatively more residents of rural areas than of urban areas; the proportion of abstainers is greatest in the southern and mountain states. Although the reasons for abstention vary, a substantial majority of abstainers cite similar reasons, ranging from moral prohibition to the desire to avoid alcohol-related problems to the fact that they socialize with people who do not drink.

Knupfer (1989) noted a relationship between social class and consumption. Among the upper classes in the US, abstention is rare, particularly among males; only 5% of upper-class males and 9% of upper-class females abstain. Among the lower classes, 35% of males and 57% of females abstain. At the same time, the category of "frequent light to moderately heavy" drinkers includes nearly 70% of both upper-class men and upper-class women, but only one-third of lower-class men and less than 20% of lower-class women.

Consumption of alcohol has increased in Europe during the past three decades. What makes the US unique is that its abstaining population has held relatively constant at more than 30%, while in Europe, abstention has dropped to a low level. Canada has an abstention rate of 15 to 20%, probably the world's second highest. Abstention rates are no more than 10% in Italy, and as low as 8% in Great Britain and 5% in West Germany. In addition to the third of the US population who do not drink, another 15% say they drink less than once a month, meaning that nearly one-half of the adults in the US consume little or no alcohol (Clark, 1991). The historical increase in per capita consumption in the US is attributed not to an increase in the proportion of drinkers (as in Europe), but to an increase in the average consumption per drinker. Although the US is near the world median in per-capita alcohol consumption, consumption per drinker is probably about the highest in the world (Room, 1983).

The aggregate consumption distribution

The French epidemiologist Ledermann (1964) was the first to empirically demonstrate a continuous unimodal (one-peak) distribution of alcohol consumption. Previously, popular belief held that drinkers fell into two groups: those who drink safely and acceptably, and those who drink heavily and dependently (i.e., alcoholics). In the years since his early work, Ledermann's statistical assumptions about the distribution have been criticized (Skog, 1985; Duffy, 1986; Tan, Lemmens & Koning, 1990). However, a continuous unimodal distribution of consumption is generally accepted.

Surveys of self-reported drinking over time and across populations have found that distributions of average daily consumption are skewed sharply to the right, with the majority of the population falling at or near zero. As one moves from the mode (the most common consumption level) to the right, fewer and fewer people are represented at any point in the distribution, and the curve slopes downward. At the extreme end of the distribution are the heaviest drinkers. The curve ends at the natural physiological limit of consumption, above which a person would be likely to die.

One mathematical form that appears to describe the empirically observed distribution of consumption is the lognormal probability-density function (the distribution of a random variable whose logarithm is normally distributed). The values in this distribution are necessarily positive. The function is defined in terms of the mean (μ) and standard deviation (σ) of this distribution. The lognormal distribution has proven useful for fitting data describing a wide range of natural phenomena, in fields ranging from biology to meteorology to economics (Crow & Shimizu, 1988). Following work by Larsen (1969), the US Environmental Protection Agency has based air pollution standards on lognormal distributions. Lognormal distributions have been applied to such diverse phenomena as labor turnover (McLean, 1976), the metal content of rock chips (Krige, 1966), insurance claims (Seal, 1969), and economic variables, such as income (Aitchison & Brown, 1957) and consumer demand (Crouch & Oglesby, 1978).

Figure 2.1 illustrates a right-skewed continuous distribution of consumption; the vertical axis represents the percentage of drinkers at each consumption level, and the horizontal axis represents mean daily consumption in ounces of absolute ethanol. This curve has a unique mean and standard deviation, and its shape will change as either or both of these parameters changes. The four consumption classes used in *SimCom*, as described above, are indicated by shading of segments of the curve. The number of people in each class can be calculated by integrating between the

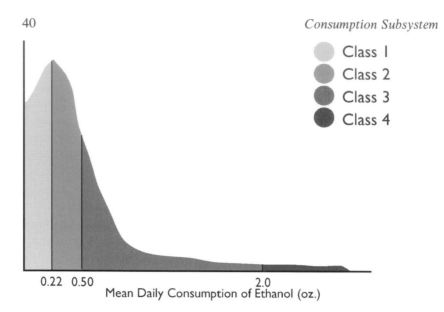

Figure 2.1 Four alcohol consumption classes within a continuous distribution.

upper and lower consumption limits of the class.

The rationale for a skewed distribution of consumption (rather than a normal or bell-shaped distribution) is that the individual has limited freedom of choice about consumption. Ledermann (1964) argued that if individuals were totally free, their consumption would in all likelihood follow a normal (Gaussian) distribution. Following this line of reasoning, Skog (1982) reached the following conclusion:

> Instead of developing their drinking habits freely and independently of the environment, individuals are socialized into a drinking pattern which to a large degree is dependent on the norms and traditions of the environment. This social pressure has as [its] result that the process of development will behave as a series of proportionally acting impulses, and that the changes in the consumption of the individuals always remain proportional to the consumption at a previous point in time. When consumption develops this way, the individuals will gradually become lognormally distributed.

While arguing against Ledermann's particular statistical assumptions, Skog (1985) elaborated on the proposition of a unimodal distribution, asserting that a population's aggregate consumption changes tend to be reflected at all consumption levels and can be tracked as the mean (average) per capita consumption of absolute ethanol. Skog contends that mean consumption has a sociocultural content far beyond its algebraic definition as the arithmetic mean of individual consumption levels. If society is viewed as an interlinked web of networks, from small, intimate ones to larger and larger ones, behavioral change in one part of a network is likely to have an effect that spreads outward. A change in mean consumption indicates a change in consumption by drinkers at all levels, "moving in concert" up or down the consumption scale (Skog, 1985).

Skog (1985) proposed not only that all drinkers change their consumption in the same general direction, but that with a change in mean population consumption, drinkers at all levels change their consumption to a degree roughly proportional to their existing consumption levels (i.e., in a manner similar to that predicted by the Weber–Fechner law of proportionate effects). Skog (1985) argued that a change in average daily alcohol consumption of 0.1 oz. (or 2.957 ml) would be more significant for a light drinker than for a heavy drinker. If daily consumption were increasing throughout a given population, therefore, heavy drinkers would be likely to increase their consumption by greater amounts than light drinkers.

See a recent analyses by Lemmons (1995) who found that a slight change in the overall consumption distribution can have a large effect on mortality but that estimates of changes in the right tail of the distributions can have considerable room for error.

Alcohol consumption is dynamic

As a dynamic system itself, the Consumption Subsystem continuously adjusts in response to both exogenous factors (outside of the subsystem) and endogenous factors (within the subsystem). Within any age group, people may change their drinking patterns in response to these factors. Movement between consumption categories can be triggered by changes in such factors as disposable income, alcohol prices, and social norms. Each consumption category can be described in terms of the net movement of people in and out of that category at any point in time. Although a person theoretically may move between any two consumption categories, he or she is most likely to move into an adjacent category. One obvious exception is that people occasionally move from one of the highest two consumption categories to total abstention. Possible and typical movements between consumption categories are illustrated in Fig. 2.2.

For each age and gender group, movement between consumption categories can be governed by factors external to the Consumption Subsystem such as:

(1) Personal income (consumption of each of the three types of alcoholic beverage is uniquely sensitive to income changes).

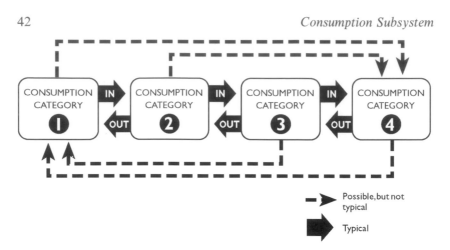

Figure 2.2 Movement of population between consumption categories.

(2) Retail price of beer, wine, and spirits.
(3) The retail and social availability of beer, wine, and spirits.
(4) The minimum age for purchase (or drinking) of each of the three
     beverage types.
(5) Social norms for alcohol consumption levels and settings.

Movement between consumption categories also is influenced by the endogenous factor of prior average alcohol consumption by the community.

Income

Income has an important influence on consumption levels and on the proportion of the population that abstains from alcohol (National Institute on Drug Abuse, 1988, 1990; Hilton, 1991). As income rises, abstinence declines, and vice versa. Among those who drink, income is predictive of personal consumption levels. Income establishes one's ability to purchase alcohol, and it provides a barrier or stimulus to drinking in addition to the influences of religious values and the overall drinking environment. (For a summary of international research on the relationship between income and alcohol consumption, see Österberg, 1995.)

Price of alcohol

Alcohol consumption responds to changes in retail prices of alcoholic beverages; as price increases, consumption declines, and vice versa. The inverse relationship between price and consumption in the US is confirmed by the econometric research of Cook & Tauchen (1982), Hoadley, Fuchs & Holder (1984), and Ornstein & Hanssens (1981). Grossman, Coate & Arluck (1987) determined the differential price sensitivity of consumption for all types of alcoholic beverages by young people (16 to 21 years old). For summaries of international research on the relationship between price and alcohol consumption, see Österberg, 1995.

Physical availability of alcohol

The retail availability of alcohol influences the level of consumption. Extreme restrictions on the number of outlets can reduce the level of consumption and various indications of alcohol problems. Prohibition (both in the US and in other nations) did result in lowered consumption rates, even allowing for illegal alcohol consumption (Bruun et al., 1975; Moore & Gerstein, 1981). There is evidence that other restrictions on availability, notably strikes affecting alcohol production or retail outlets, can reduce alcohol-related problems (Bruun et al., 1975; Edwards et al., 1994). As discussed in greater detail in Chapter 3, availability of alcohol and demand for alcohol (expressed as sales) are reciprocally related; greater outlet densities are related to greater alcohol consumption and vice versa (Gruenewald, Ponicki & Holder, 1993).

Minimum drinking age

Changes in the legal minimum drinking age (i.e., the age at which one can legally purchase alcohol) can result in changes in the quantity and frequency of alcohol consumption by young people. Basing their research on national adolescent drinking studies in the US, Maisto & Rachal (1980) reported that in areas where the drinking age is higher, per capita consumption among the young is lower. Longitudinal analyses of aggregate sales have shown that sales of beer (and sometimes wine) are sensitive to changes in the drinking age (Smart, 1977; Wagenaar, 1983, 1986). In a national evaluation of the sensitivity of underage consumption to minimum drinking age, Grossman, Coate & Arluck (1987) found that a one-year increase in the legal drinking age in for each specific beverage lowers the drinking participation rate by 5.6%. O'Malley & Wagenaar (1991) found that the minimum drinking age continues to affect consumption into young adulthood, long after members of the age group are legally allowed to drink.

Ontario lowered the purchase age from 21 to 18 concurrent with the policy trend in the early 1970s in the US; thereafter Ontario experienced an increase in the incidence of alcohol-related car crashes among the young (Whitehead et al., 1975; Williams et al., 1975). Schmidt & Kornaczewski (1975) found significant increases in the number of traffic accidents among Ontario drivers 16 to 19 years old.

Bracketing in time the 1971 lowering of drinking age from 21 to 18, cross-sectional surveys of Toronto high school students were undertaken in 1968, 1970, 1972, and 1974. The proportion of students who had used alcohol at least once increased immediately before and after the age change (1970–72), but an even larger increase occurred between 1968 and 1970 (Smart & Fejer, 1975).

Apart from these high school studies, the Canadian research offers conclusions very much in the same direction as the US reports.

Social norms

Drinking is a culturally influenced behavior, reflecting perceived social encouragement or restriction of alcohol consumption. In an early empirical study, Larsen & Abu-Laban (1968) found that consumption increases or decreases depending on the extent of norms proscribing drinking or prescribing consumption limits. Skog (1980) has described drinking as a social act in which an individual's drinking habits are largely defined and determined by the drinking habits of others. He described a web of interlinked social networks, within which drinking norms define the drinking habits of individuals and between which these norms may be transferred.

A community's drinking norms may change over time as the proportion of the population belonging to religious groups with proscriptive norms changes. Different racial and ethnic groups also have distinctive patterns of consumption. For instance, surveys of Mexican-Americans in California have found that while their aggregate consumption tends to equal that for the US population as a whole, they show significant differences in abstention rates, consumption frequency, and quantity consumed per occasion. Caetano & Kaskutas (1996) found that overall, Mexican-American men and women drink less frequently but more per occasion than do men and women in the US population as a whole. Caetano (1995) and Caetano & Medina-Mora (1988) also found that in northern California, African-American and Mexican-American women have higher rates of abstention than do white women. Herd (1991) found that nearly one-half of African-American women (46%) were abstainers in 1984, compared with about one-third (34%) of white women. She reported that aggregate drinking levels for white and African-American men were nearly equal, although their drinking patterns differed across age groups, and in frequency and quantity per occasion.

Responses of consumption distributions to stimulus factors

In the dynamic Consumption Subsystem, a change in a stimulus factor (e.g., price) will result in some corresponding response in consumption. The relative size of this response can be expressed as the sensitivity, or "elasticity," of consumption to a stimulus factor. An elasticity typically is expressed in percentage terms; the elasticity is the corresponding percentage change in the dependent factor (in this case, consumption) for every 1% change in a stimulus factor. Thus, a stimulus factor's effect on consumption can be expressed by the following relationship:

$$\text{Consumption}_t = \text{Consumption}_{t-1} \times (1 + [\Delta\text{Stimulus Factor}_t \times \text{Elasticity}])$$

In this equation, current consumption (consumption at time = t) is equal to previous consumption (consumption at time = t − 1) multiplied by 1 plus the product of the percentage change (indicated by Δ) in the stimulus factor and the elasticity.

This simple equation suggests a linear and unchanging relationship between the stimulus factor and consumption; elasticity remains constant. However, in a dynamic system, one can expect relationships between stimulus factors and consumption to be non-linear and to vary over time. Figure 2.3 illustrates several possible relationships between consumption and stimulus factors. In each graph (A–F), the vertical axis is the level of alcohol consumption (for example, the per capita consumption by an age and gender group), and the horizontal axis is the level of the exogenous variable, such as alcohol price or personal income.

Graph A illustrates the case where changes in an exogenous factor have no effect on consumption. Such a factor is, by definition, not a stimulus factor. Graphs B and C illustrate a simple linear (positive or negative) association between consumption and changes in the stimulus factor. This is the type of relationship specified by the equation given above. Other possibilities exist. Graphs D and F show positive and negative non-linear associations, respectively. In these examples, consumption rises or declines rapidly over a defined range of levels of the stimulus factor, but beyond this range, the effect slows considerably (as though reaching a ceiling or lower/

A. No differential responses

B. Positive, linear association

C. Negative, linear association

D. Positive association
   (ceiling effect)

E. Exponential association
   (unlimited growth)

F. Negative (asymptotic effect)

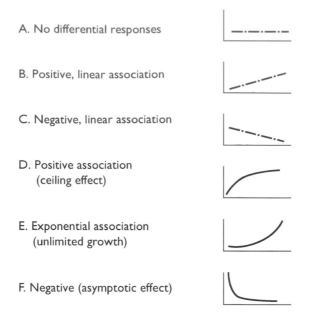

Figure 2.3 Alternative differential sensitivity between consumption and stimulus factors.

upper limit). As the limit is approached (becomes asymptotic), the effect of the exogenous factor on consumption becomes less and less, approaching (but probably never reaching) zero. Graph E illustrates a positive exponential (unlimited) relationship, where consumption increases exponentially as the stimulus factor increases linearly.

In a complex dynamic system, the elasticities of consumption to stimulus factors need not be constant, but can vary. Elasticity can be influenced by the magnitude of the change in the stimulus factor at any point in time. For example, a gradual change in alcohol price, say less than 10% per unit time, may well be absorbed by the consumer in such a way that the change in consumption represents (or looks like) a fixed elasticity. However, if the price of alcohol suddenly increases dramatically (say 20 to 50%) while other retail prices and income remain relatively constant, then the fixed elasticity may not account for the response of consumption, even allowing for consumer substitution of lower-priced brands for higher-priced ones.

Figure 2.4 illustrates a possible dynamic elasticity, in this case a hy-

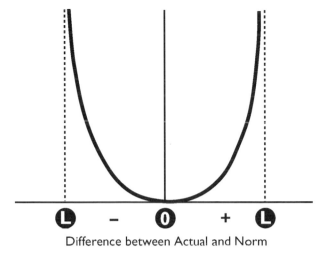

Difference between Actual and Norm

Figure 2.4 Relationship of elasticity to difference between norm and actual per capita consumption level.

pothesized relationship between the actual average level of alcohol consumption and the socially acceptable level. In this illustration, the greater the distance between the acceptable and actual consumption levels, the greater the social pressure on actual consumption to shift towards the socially accepted level. In Fig. 2.4, this varying elasticity is illustrated as a standard parabola. The difference between the socially acceptable per capita consumption level and actual per capita consumption is shown on the horizontal axis as ranging between limits (L). At the midpoint (0), the actual and accepted levels of consumption are equal. As the difference between the socially acceptable and actual levels increases – either positively (norm > actual) or negatively (norm < actual) – the elasticity increases, representing greater pressure on actual consumption to change in the direction of the socially acceptable level. As the gap between the socially acceptable and actual consumption levels decreases (the difference approaches 0), the elasticity decreases, representing less pressure for consumption to change.

Influence of the drinking environment on consumption

Drinking environment has an important influence on drinking patterns, with respect not only to quantity and frequency of alcohol consumption, but also to levels of abstinence. For example, Knupfer & Room (1970) and Hilton (1991) found that if the social situations in which people participate do not involve alcohol, people are less likely to drink alcohol to be sociable. In other words, the "drier" the social environment, the greater the likelihood of abstinence. The influence of the social environment on consumption patterns may be considered at a micro-level (e.g., within a small group or an extended family in a community); however, the overall community drinking environment is expected to have a larger influence.

The more prominent drinking is in community life (i.e., the 'wetter" the social environment), the lower the abstinence rates are likely to be across age and gender groups. Conversely, the less prominent drinking is, the higher the abstinence rates are likely to be. In other words, the percentage of the population that abstains depends in part on the relative importance of drinking within the community in general, as indicated by the average alcohol consumption in the community, which can be considered the 'expected" consumption. The influence of the community drinking environment on any individual or group within the community can be expressed as the distance of that individual's or group's consumption from the expected level: the greater this distance, the stronger the influence. Similarly, the drinking pattern of the community as a whole is influenced by the distance between community consumption and the 'expected" consumption based on the larger social context (i.e., regional or national patterns). Highly "dry" or highly "wet" alcohol environments will be under more pressure to move towards the expected consumption level than environments where consumption is closer to the expected level.

The hypothesized influence of drinking environment on community consumption is illustrated in Fig. 2.5. In this example, national per capita consumption of alcohol is used as a point of reference for consumption in community systems. The greater the influence of national social values and the greater distance of community consumption from the national norm, the greater the pressure on the community to move toward the national consumption norm. Figure 2.5 illustrates a plot of national per capita consumption and consumption in two hypothetical communities, X and Y, over a 20–year period. At time A, a considerable gap exists between consumption levels for community X and the country; this large difference would be expected to create considerable pressure on community X to move toward the country norm (e.g., to increase per capita consumption and lower the percentage of abstainers). At time B, the gap between country and community consumption has narrowed, as a result of increasing consumption in community X and decreasing consumption nationally;

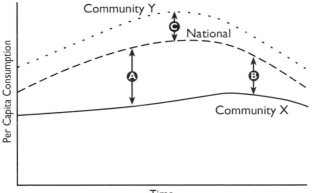

Figure 2.5 Differences in national per capita and community alcohol consumption levels.

thus, pressure to move toward the country norm would be less than at point A. In this example, at time C, consumption in community Y is higher than the norm for the nation, creating pressure to decrease consumption (e.g., to lower per capita consumption and increase the number of abstainers).

Drinks per occasion, impairment, and blood alcohol concentration

To this point, consumption has been discussed in terms of average quantity frequency or per capita consumption over some time period. However, any measure of average consumption is based on the aggregate of a variety of drinking patterns. An especially important aspect of variation in drinking patterns is the amount of alcohol consumed during one drinking period or event, often measured as "drinks per occasion" (DPO), defined as the number of drinks consumed during each drinking event. Event drinking contributes most importantly to acute alcohol-involved problems, whereas average consumption is related to the risk of chronic health problems from long term exposure to ethanol. Prevention interventions that seek to reduce the amount of alcohol consumed per drinking occasion are designed to reduce the blood alcohol concentration, or impairment, and thus to lower the risk of acute events in the moment; they may not specifically be designed to reduce average per capita consumption.

Drinks per occasion can be represented as a distribution from 0 to some large number (e.g., 15 or 20), associated with each consumption class for

Table 2.2. *Drinks per occasion by consumption class*

	Total drinks consumed at one occasion									
Class	1	2	3	4	5	6	7	8	9	10+
1										
2										
3										
4										

each age and gender group. For example, Table 2.2 illustrates an 11–interval distribution of DPO from 0 to 10+ drinks, using four consumption classes (as used in *SimCom*). One such matrix would be created to represent each age and gender group. Each cell in the matrix would contain the number or percentage of people in the consumption class who fall into the applicable DPO column. Alternatively, individual DPO values beyond ten drinks could be specified, resulting in more matrix columns, or DPO categories could be combined, resulting in fewer matrix columns.

Instead of being displayed as a matrix, the range of DPO could be described by a functional form based on empirical data. For example, based on analysis of consumption surveys in the US, the following functional form was selected to best represent the distribution of DPO over all gender and age groups in *SimCom*:

$$\ln y = a + bx + c\sqrt{x} \quad \text{or} \quad y = e^{(a + bx + c\sqrt{x})}$$

where y = percentage of people who consume X drinks per occasion, x = the average or expected number of drinks per occasion, e = the base of the natural system of logarithms, and a, b, and c are empirically determined parameters that vary across age and gender groups.

DPO distributions provide the basis for estimating levels of alcohol impairment and thus the risk of alcohol-involved problems, such as alcohol-involved traffic crashes or alcohol-involved non-traffic-related injuries or fatalities. Blood alcohol concentration (BAC) can be used as a surrogate for the level of impairment. The BAC resulting from a given number of number of drinks consumed is a function of the individual's age, weight, and alcohol absorption rate, which depends on the amount of food consumed and the time over which alcohol is consumed. Using an average expected body weight for an age and gender group, an expected BAC per drinks consumed at one occasion can be derived, as shown in Table 2.3

(calculated according to the formula of Fisher, Simpson & Kuper, 1987). Of course food consumption which affects the rate of alcohol absorption can alter the maximum BAC achieved. The ranges of BAC for each age and gender group were derived by taking the mean weight for the group plus or minus one standard deviation. BAC values derived from the ranges in Table 2.3 can be used to convert any set of mean drinks per occasion (e.g., from Table 2.2) into an expected BAC value. This allows the risk of acute alcohol-involved problems (e.g., crashes or injuries) to be estimated for each consumption group by age and gender.

Thus, the Consumption Subsystem is composed of distributions of average consumption across the drinking population, as well as distributions of DPO associated with consumption groups, where the consumption groups are defined segments of the continuous consumption distribution (as shown in Fig. 2.1).

Interaction with other subsystems

As a complex adaptive system, the Consumption Subsystem is continuously adjusting in response to changing forces both within and outside of the subsystem. The distribution of average alcohol consumption is altered by external forces, such as price of alcohol, personal income, retail availability of alcohol, and social norms related to alcohol use, as well as by structures and factors within the subsystem, such as changes in age and gender distributions, and natural, unpredictable (stochastic or probabilistic) shifts in distributions internal to the subsystem. The distribution of DPO responds to changes in the same factors, as well as to changes in the distribution of average consumption and to purposeful prevention interventions targeting the DPO distribution, such as server training and regulation of drink prices at bars or pubs.

Thus, the Consumption Subsystem is affected by the Retail Sales and Social Norms subsystems, and by the exogenous factors of economic trends and population growth and decline. In turn, the Consumption Subsystem provides inputs into the Retail Sales, Social Norms, Legal Sanctions, and Social, Economic, and Health Consequences subsystems. (These interactions are illustrated in Chapter 1, Fig. 1.3.)

Given the dynamic nature of the Consumption Subsystem, it is not difficult to see that efforts to alter the drinking of specific targeted individuals are unlikely to reduce aggregate community alcohol problems. Responding to internal and external forces, the Consumption Subsystem not only adjusts to naturally occurring changes, but resists purposeful efforts

Table 2.3. BAC range estimated by age and gender from consumption at one occasion

Age	Mean	SD	Number of Drinks (Milliliters of Ethanol)									
			1 (14.787)	2 (29.574)	3 (44.361)	4 (59.148)	5 (73.935)	6 (88.722)	7 (103.509)	8 (118.296)	9 (133.083)	10 (147.870)
Males												
18–20	165	30	0.02–0.03	0.04–0.06	0.06–0.09	0.08–0.12	0.11–0.15	0.13–0.18	0.15–0.21	0.17–0.24	0.19–0.27	0.21–0.30
21–25	167	31	0.02–0.03	0.04–0.06	0.06–0.09	0.08–0.12	0.10–0.15	0.12–0.18	0.15–0.21	0.17–0.24	0.19–0.27	0.21–0.30
26–34	176	35	0.02–0.03	0.04–0.06	0.06–0.09	0.08–0.12	0.10–0.15	0.12–0.17	0.14–0.20	0.16–0.23	0.18–0.26	0.19–0.29
35–49	177	30	0.02–0.03	0.04–0.06	0.06–0.08	0.08–0.11	0.10–0.14	0.12–0.17	0.14–0.20	0.16–0.22	0.18–0.25	0.20–0.28
50–64	171	30	0.02–0.03	0.04–0.06	0.06–0.09	0.08–0.12	0.10–0.15	0.12–0.17	0.14–0.20	0.16–0.23	0.18–0.26	0.20–0.29
65+	164	27	0.02–0.03	0.04–0.06	0.06–0.09	0.09–0.12	0.11–0.15	0.13–0.18	0.15–0.21	0.17–0.24	0.19–0.27	0.22–0.30
Females												
18–20	132	27	0.03–0.05	0.06–0.09	0.09–0.14	0.12–0.19	0.16–0.24	0.19–0.28	0.22–0.33	0.25–0.38	0.28–0.42	0.31–0.47
21–25	133	28	0.03–0.05	0.06–0.09	0.09–0.14	0.12–0.19	0.15–0.24	0.18–0.28	0.21–0.33	0.25–0.38	0.28–0.42	0.31–0.47
26–34	140	32	0.03–0.05	0.06–0.09	0.09–0.14	0.11–0.18	0.14–0.23	0.17–0.27	0.20–0.32	0.23–0.37	0.26–0.41	0.29–0.46
35–49	148	35	0.03–0.04	0.05–0.09	0.08–0.13	0.11–0.17	0.14–0.22	0.16–0.26	0.19–0.31	0.22–0.35	0.24–0.39	0.27–0.44
50–64	149	33	0.03–0.04	0.05–0.09	0.08–0.13	0.11–0.17	0.14–0.21	0.16–0.26	0.19–0.30	0.22–0.34	0.24–0.38	0.27–0.43
65+	146	29	0.03–0.04	0.06–0.08	0.08–0.13	0.11–0.17	0.14–0.21	0.17–0.25	0.20–0.30	0.23–0.34	0.25–0.38	0.28–0.42

Sources:
1. *Vital Statistics* for weight.
2. Calculation of BAC by gender, weight, number of drinks, and time converted from Fisher, Simpson & Kuper (1987).

by prevention programs to disturb the subsystem's natural dynamics. The subsystem's adaptive behavior can counteract prevention interventions based on targeting individual behavior and block their long-term effectiveness.

3

Retail Sales Subsystem: alcohol availability and promotion

Introduction

Alcohol is made available to consumers through the Retail Sales Subsystem. Alcohol may be legally or illegally produced. It is produced and distributed by a beverage industry (which may or may not be located within the community system) and sold in a variety of forms and quantities, through several types of retail outlets. Within the Retail Sales Subsystem, two key factors – retail availability and consumer demand for alcohol – interact to determine the level of retail sales of alcohol in a community, which is equivalent to the overall level of consumption.

In industrialized countries, the Retail Sales Subsystem is affected by the formal licensing and regulation of retail alcohol outlets. Restraints and restrictions on retail availability of alcohol, including zoning and other local regulation of alcohol outlets as businesses, are inputs to the Retail Sales Subsystem from the Formal Regulation and Control Subsystem. Even if, as in non-industrialized communities, alcohol is available through indigenous private production and sale, rather than formally licensed shops or bars and restaurants, such transactions still constitute a Retail Sales Subsystem.

The Retail Sales Subsystem for alcohol is a part of the community's overall retail marketplace. As part of the economic structure of a community, outlets for the sale of alcohol are influenced by the same types of economic factors that influence retail outlets for other non-durable (consumable or disposable) goods, such as food, clothing, motion pictures, cosmetics, and automobiles. The Retail Sales Subsystem for alcohol is strongly influenced by overall community economic factors, such as the strength or weakness of the local economy, corporate profitability, inflation, personal income, and consumer demand for retail goods and services in general (not only for alcohol). For example, the numbers of retail outlets

54

that sell goods and services in addition to alcohol (such as restaurants or grocery stores) are more strongly influenced by the demand for these types of general retail establishments than by the single demand for alcohol outlets. Also, the affordability of alcohol to the consumer depends not only on retail price, but on personal income and the cost of alcohol relative to the costs of other goods and services. Thus, general economic forces are exogenous factors that serve as inputs to the Retail Sales Subsystem.

The Retail Sales Subsystem also is affected by the particular economic attributes of alcohol sales, such as price competition and the effects of added national and regional/local alcohol taxes. The retail price of alcohol is the sum of the wholesale price (including manufacturers' and distributors' costs), taxes, and the retailers' costs and profit. Consumer demand for alcohol is a function of consumer preferences and perceived needs. In addition, retailers of alcohol seek to influence the demand for alcohol through promotion and marketing, competitive pricing, and the location and convenience of alcohol outlets. Finally, research has shown that the relationship between retail availability of alcohol and consumer demand for alcohol is reciprocal: not only does demand influence availability, but availability influences demand.

This chapter first defines possible types of retail outlets for alcohol and explains some basic economic principles affecting retail sales. It also describes the effects of formal regulation and of general economic forces on the Retail Sales Subsystem. It then describes the complex ways in which availability, price, and demand interact to determine retail sales of alcohol, and thus consumption.

Retail sales outlets for alcohol and the influence of formal regulation on outlet types

Retail outlets selling alcohol within a culture where alcohol sales are legal and regulated by the government can be simply categorized as "on-premises" or "off-premises" establishments. On-premises establishments sell alcohol for consumption on the outlets' own premises; examples are bars, pubs, and restaurants. Off-premises establishments sell alcohol in containers for consumption at other locations; examples are wine shops, liquor stores, mini-markets, and grocery stores. If the law permits, a retail establishment may be licensed for both on-premises and off-premises sales. For example, a bar might sell spirits for off-premises consumption, or a general store might sell beer for on-premises consumption. If alcohol is not formally regulated by the government, then informal outlets of alcohol may develop in response to demand. See discussion by Marshall & Marshall (1990) about the Pacific Island of Moen in Truk, Federated State of Micronesia.

Alcohol outlets can be further categorized as "general-purpose" or "special-purpose" establishments. General-purpose, off-premises outlets are general stores that sell goods in addition to alcohol, such as grocery or food stores, convenience stores, drug stores, and gasoline stations. Special-purpose, off-premises outlets are stores that primarily sell alcoholic beverages, such as publicly or privately owned liquor stores. The most common general-purpose, on-premises outlets are restaurants, which primarily sell food for consumption on the premises. Special-purpose, on-premises outlets are bars or pubs, which primarily sell alcoholic beverages for consumption on the premises and which may or may not offer food as a secondary sales option.

The Retail Sales Subsystem potentially can include all the possible combinations of beverage type (beer, wine, or distilled spirits) and retail establishment type (general or special purpose) shown in Table 3.1. However, depending on the laws governing alcohol sales and the practical reality of consumer demand, some of these types of establishments may be prohibited, or unlikely, to exist in a given community within a specific country. For example, in California (USA), which permits privately licensed outlets, wine production is an important industry, and wine specialty stores (type D) are popular. However, because outlets usually must sell multiple beverage types in order to survive economically, establishment types A, B, C, E, and F are unlikely in California. In North Carolina (USA), spirits are available only in state monopoly stores (type F); establishment types E, I, J, K, and L do not exist. Until 1978, a portion of type M (restaurants selling spirits along with beer and wine) did not exist in North Carolina. The other portion of type M (privately licensed stores, such as grocery stores or liquor stores, selling spirits along with beer and wine) still is not permitted. In the Nordic Countries of Sweden, Norway, and Finland, a public monopoly for off-premise retail sales of wine, spirits, and higher alcohol content beer exists (Kortteinen, 1989).

Price and the demand–supply relationship

In a rational model of the retail firm (as discussed by Betancourt & Gautschi, 1988), the firm desires to set a price that represents its cost for the goods (wholesale cost) plus a maximal profit. Two factors act to restrain

Table 3.1. *Alcohol establishments types*

	General Purpose	Special Purpose
Beer only	A	B
Wine only	C	D
Spirits only	E	F
Beer and wine	G	H
Beer and spirits	I	J
Wine and spirits	K	L
All beverages	M	N

maximization of profit – competition and consumer demand. Thus, the price a retailer sets for a product is a function of at least three factors:

(1) The cost of the product, including the cost of making the product available to the consumer.
(2) The price at which the consumer can purchase the product at another retail establishment at equal total cost (i.e., the product's price plus the cost to acquire it, such as travel costs and time spent).
(3) Consumer demand for the product, which affects the price the consumer is willing to pay.

The relationship between demand and supply is one of the foundations of economics. The supply of goods is driven by consumer demand. The consumer identifies a need or desire for a product or service and seeks a source to meet this need, and the supplier responds to the demand. By this elementary proposition, supply depends totally on demand and thus is a passive participant in the demand–supply relationship. Such a relationship may be further specified by demand and supply curves, as shown in Fig. 3.1. The supply curve, S, shows the relationship between the retail price of a product and the quantity that producers are willing (i.e., economically stimulated) to sell. As price increases, producers are willing to sell more and more of a product. The demand curve, D, shows the relationship between retail price of a product and the quantity that consumers will purchase. As price increases, consumers will purchase less (i.e., demand less) of the goods. When S and D curves are plotted together, their intersection (shown as P_0, Q_0) represents the price at which demand and supply are in equilibrium – the point where consumers and producers "agree" on a price and available quantity of a product.

According to this simple economic principle, the market sets the price. When more of a product is produced than consumers are willing to

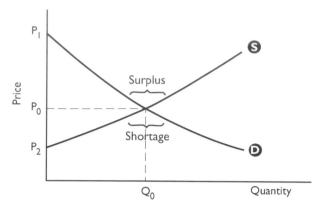

Figure 3.1 Demand and supply curves.

purchase, a surplus is created, and prices are expected to decrease. When demand exceeds the supply of the product, the price is expected to rise in response to demand. For example, when the automobile manufacturer Mazda introduced the Miata sports car to the US market during 1989–90, the cars were unexpectedly popular; not enough cars were produced to meet demand, so the selling price rose despite the manufacturer's efforts to maintain a set price. According to traditional price-action theory (as discussed by Nooteboom, Kleijweg & Thurik, 1988), prices adjust in proportion to excess demand or supply until a set of prices is reached that clears the market of excess demand or capacity. If equilibrium between supply and demand is maintained, prices adjust to marginal costs. (For further discussion of the demand–supply relationship, see Pindyck & Rubinfeld, 1989.)

In most free-market economies, however, the relationship between supply and demand is more complicated, because sources of retail supply have developed means to stimulate demand. That is, markets of goods and services have become less passive in the demand–supply relationship. Figure 3.2 shows the influence of marketing efforts on the demand–supply relationship. The cause-and-effect relationship between demand and supply is complicated by the addition of a feedback loop reflecting the effects of marketing. Alcohol producers and retail suppliers, like their counterparts in other retail goods, recognize the value of promotion and advertising to consumer demand. While some countries limit or ban alcohol advertising of specific types or for specific beverages, for example in Sweden, Norway, and Finland, whenever possible there is a clear economic incentive to market alcoholic products. One purpose of advertising is to

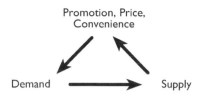

Figure 3.2 The reciprocal interaction of supply and demand.

differentiate and increase the sale of specific brands. In addition, alcohol advertising can assist in normalizing drinking. See discussion by Casswell (1995) and Chapter 5.

In marketing theory, efforts to stimulate demand are referred to as the "three Ps" – price, promotion, and place. Pricing, advertising, and location in terms of customer convenience (which depends on the number of retail sources and their distances from customers) are determined by the sources of supply.

Although demand generally stimulates supply, supply also can stabilize demand. If demand is high, but supply is insufficient or non-existent, then demand can diminish or stabilize. Thus, short supply can act as a damper on demand.

Alcoholic beverages behave in the market in the same ways as other goods: as prices decline or incomes increase, alcohol sales tend to increase, and as prices increase or incomes decline, alcohol sales tend to decrease. "Price elasticity" is the amount of change in demand for goods (usually expressed as a percent change in retail purchases) in response to a 1% change in price. Studies from a number of countries have estimated the elasticity of alcohol sales to changes in price and income (e.g., Cook & Tauchen, 1982; Levy & Sheflin, 1983, Ornstein & Levy, 1983; Saffer & Grossman, 1987; Leung & Phelps, 1993). International research on price and income has been summarized by Österberg (1995).

Factors affecting the number and density of alcohol retail sales outlets

A basic tenet of economics is that the numbers and locations of a specific type of retail establishment depend on the size and density of the population of potential consumers. Each type of business has a population threshold – the smallest market area capable of supporting the smallest economically feasible establishment of its type. For instance, if the population threshold is 2500 for restaurants and 5000 for dry cleaners, one might expect a community with a population of 3000 to have a restaurant but not a dry cleaner. One might use this approach to estimate the number of a particular type of establishment needed to serve consumer demand per unit of population, such as the number of bars and restaurants needed per 1000 people. Similarly, one could calculate the minimum population an area must have for a singles bar to be economically viable.

In addition, the factors of location, distance, and convenience interact to shape both the behavior of consumers and the development of retail outlets. According to economic theory, consumers purchasing goods that yield satisfaction will minimize the cost (and time) to attain the goods through their choice of sales locations and quantities of goods (Betancourt & Gautschi, 1988). The number of alcohol outlets in a community and their geographical relationships also are influenced by other population centers; in general, larger population centers attract business (hence retail establishments) away from smaller population clusters (Berry, 1968). The Retail Sales Subsystem produces the number and distribution of outlets needed to serve a specific consumer demand.

Researchers have confirmed that population and personal income are important factors influencing the number and density of retail establishments. For example, Lakshmanan & Hansen (1965) found the size and number of retail establishments to be related to the aggregate purchasing power of consumers. Clements (1978) found population to be the strongest predictor of retail trade patterns. Markin (1974) concluded that income and population are the two major determinants of consumption of goods and services in retail markets.

One factor that particularly influences the number of retail alcohol outlets is tourism. In a community that attracts many non-resident visitors, such as a beach or seaside community or a popular tourist center, alcohol consumption by visitors can increase the demand for retail alcohol outlets. In constructing models of alcohol demand, both Nelson (1988) and Ornstein & Hanssens (1985) found tourism to be a strong predictor of alcohol demand (after price and income). Tourism is more likely to increase the demand for on-premises establishments than for off-premises ones.

The general business climate, which reflects the potential profitability of economic investment, also has an important influence on number and density of retail outlets. The willingness of a current or potential business owner to risk capital in a retail outlet depends on whether he or she believes the investment can be profitable.

These factors have different effects on the different types of retail alcohol outlets. For example, because alcohol sale is the primary function of bars or pubs, their number increases or decreases with the demand for alcohol in the community. As total alcohol consumption rises (all other factors being equal), the number of bars is likely to rise; as total consumption decreases, the number of bars decreases. In contrast, because restaurants, grocery stores, and gasoline stations sell goods and services in addition to alcohol, their numbers are more influenced by general consumer demand. Populations with higher per capita income will support more alcohol-selling restaurants. A restaurant selling alcohol may fulfill some of the consumption-driven demand for an on-premises establishment and thus supplant some of the demand for a bar. Thus, the number of bars can be a function of both the overall level of alcohol consumption and the number of restaurants selling alcohol which can fulfill consumer demand for alcohol in public establishments.

The number of general stores in a community depends on the number of stores per capita that the community can support, and thus may fluctuate with the health of the local economy. If the local retail economy is weak, the density of general stores may decrease as competition between stores becomes more intense and the profitability of general stores decreases. The business climate may discourage the opening of new general-purpose establishments even when they appear warranted by population growth.

The demand for liquor stores (selling all types of beverages or specific combinations of beverages) is driven by the demand for off-premises alcohol availability, which depends on the level of alcohol consumption in the community. As total consumption rises (or falls), the number of liquor stores is expected to rise (or fall). However, some of the demand for off-premises alcohol availability may be met by general stores selling alcohol. Thus, the number of liquor stores depends on both the level of consumption and the number of general stores selling alcohol.

The reciprocal relationship between retail availability and consumption

Our understanding of the interaction between the Retail Sales Subsystem and the Consumption Subsystem is based on research that demonstrates a reciprocal relationship between availability and consumption of alcohol. According to Ornstein & Hanssens (1985) for the US and Mäkelä, Österberg & Sulkunen (1991) in Finland, the number and density of retail alcohol outlets clearly are responses to the demand for alcoholic beverages. Using data from all 50 US states in a time-series design, Gruenewald, Ponicki & Holder (1993) showed that outlet densities change in response to changes in consumption level (i.e., demand); and, conversely, increased consumption results in pressure for increased alcohol outlet densities.

Other studies had confirmed the former relationship – increased density of alcohol retail outlets increases consumer convenience, thereby increasing alcohol sales and consumption (Parker, Wolz & Harford, 1978; Harford et al., 1979; Colon, Cutter & Jones 1982). In the US, studies at the county level (Rush, Steinberg & Brook, 1986; Gliksman & Rush, 1986) and city level (Watts & Rabow, 1983) have demonstrated stable and statistically significant effects of outlet densities on consumption. In an analysis of alcohol sales data and indicators of alcohol availability in Great Britain, Godfrey (1988) found evidence for a reciprocal relationship between retail alcohol outlet densities and consumption of spirits, wine, and beer.

Further evidence for the influence of alcohol availability on consumption comes from cases where strikes of retail sales workers or production workers caused sudden reductions in alcohol availability. For example, Mäkelä (1980) found that during a strike in 1972 that closed Finnish liquor stores for five weeks, overall alcohol consumption decreased by about 30%. Although bars and restaurants continued to operate during the strike, arrests for public drunkenness declined by 50%, arrests for drinking and driving declined by 10 to 15%, and cases of assault and battery declined by as much as 25%.

In 1912, Iceland became the first country in Europe to implement total prohibition of alcohol. Spirits later were legalized, but beer continued to be banned until 1989. Olafsdottir[1] found that when beer was legalized, men added consumption of beer to their total consumption of alcohol, but women substituted beer for wine and spirits.

The types of retail outlets through which a specific type of alcoholic beverage is available can influence its consumption. Blose & Holder (1987) and Holder & Blose (1987) found that after distilled spirits were made available in on-premises establishments in one US state, North Carolina, both consumption and alcohol-involved driving crashes increased. After a state monopoly on off-premises sale of alcohol was eliminated in several US states, overall alcohol consumption increased (Holder & Wagenaar, 1990; Wagenaar & Holder, 1991, 1995).

Interaction with other subsystems

As a complex adaptive system, the Retail Sales Subsystem adjusts to changes in the social and economic environment in which it exists. In an

1 Personal communication: H. Olafsdottir. First effects of beer legalization on drinking habits. Paper presented at Alcohol Policy and Social Change Conference, Norway, September, 1990.

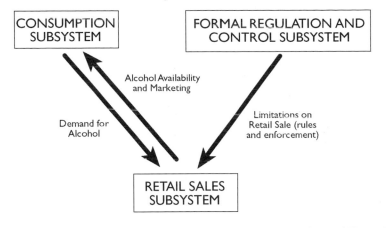

Figure 3.3 The interaction of Retail Sales with Consumption and Formal Regulation and Control Subsystems.

open market economy, as demand for alcohol increases, numbers of outlets (off-premises, on-premises, or both) are likely to increase. In addition, the number of alcohol retail outlets is influenced by general economic forces in the community system, especially in the case of outlets that sell alcohol along with other products. In turn, the demand for alcohol is influenced by its overall level of retail availability, as well as by price, convenience of purchase, and promotional marketing. This reciprocal relationship between retail availability of alcohol products and demand for them results in a dynamic relationship between the Retail Sales Subsystem and the Consumption Subsystem.

The retail availability of alcohol is governed and, in some cases, limited by rules and regulations concerning the sale of alcohol and their enforcement. In most industrialized countries, formal laws restricting alcohol wholesale and retail sales have been a central part of public policy concerning alcohol availability (Kortteinen, 1989; Edwards, et al., 1994). Within the community system, these rules, regulations, and enforcement are the domain of the Formal Regulation and Control Subsystem. The effective regulations concerning alcohol sale (i.e., formal law and the extent to which it is enforced) are inputs into the Retail Sales Subsystem from the Formal Regulation and Control Subsystem.

Figure 3.3 illustrates the interactions of the Retail Sales Subsystem with the Consumption Subsystem and the Formal Regulation and Control Subsystem.

4

Formal Regulation and Control Subsystem: rules, administration, and enforcement

Introduction

The function of the Formal Regulation and Control Subsystem is to place limits on the physical and economic availability of alcoholic beverages. Most societies establish rules and controls governing the sale and availability of alcohol. In industrialized societies, these take the form of formal laws and regulations. In fact, alcohol may be, on average, the most regulated of all legal retail products. Formal regulations typically cover the production, import, wholesale distribution, and retail sales of alcohol. The government may hold a monopoly on wholesale or retail sales of alcohol. If alcohol production and retail sales are in the hands of private corporations and individuals, these activities usually are subject to licensing and regulation.

Physical availability of alcohol may be limited through regulations controlling: the forms in which alcohol can be sold; the types, numbers, densities, and locations of retail outlets; the hours and days of the week retail sales are allowed; the minimum age to purchase or drink alcohol; serving practices; the potential liability of those serving alcohol; and the social accessibility of alcohol. Economic availability of alcohol may be regulated through taxation of alcohol sales, alcohol price restrictions and controls, and restrictions on the promotion and advertising of alcohol.

Formal regulations are publicly codified statements of societal values. Thus, the Formal Regulation and Control Subsystem is influenced by the Social Norms Subsystem, which reflects social expectations related to the use of alcohol and the community's level of concern about alcohol-involved problems. Together, the extent of formal law regulating alcohol sales and the level of enforcement of these laws establish the degree of constraint on the retail availability of alcohol to the consumer (through the Retail Sales Subsystem). If there is little or no legal regulation of alcohol sales or consumption, or if such laws exist but are not enforced, then retail sales of alcohol are effectively unrestrained, and retail availability of alcohol is determined by consumer demand (as described in Chapter 3).

This chapter explains the rationale underlying formal regulation of alcohol sales and describes the various means by which societies regulate the physical and economic availability of alcohol. As a specific example, regulation of alcohol sales in the US is described in more detail.

The rationale for regulation of alcohol sales

Three basic assumptions underlie a society's decision to regulate alcohol sales:

(1) A high level of consumption can result in high levels of alcohol-involved problems.
(2) If alcohol consumption is allowed to seek its natural level (unfettered by governmental restraint), it can stabilize at a level that the society considers unacceptably high.
(3) Restrictions on the alcohol supply can alter demand for (and consumption of) alcohol.

An argument sometimes offered against regulation of alcohol availability is that alcohol-involved problems are caused only by a small number of heavy drinkers, as a result of their alcohol dependence or addiction. These individuals will, so this conventional wisdom goes, obtain alcohol no matter what the difficulty or restrictions. However, research has demonstrated two flaws in this counter-argument:

(1) In any society, the majority of alcohol-involved problems are caused by drinkers who are not dependent drinkers.
(2) Alcohol-involved problems, including those caused by dependent drinkers, are in fact affected by changes in alcohol supply (see, for example, the relationship between alcohol, price, and chronic alcohol problems in Cook & Tauchen, 1982).

Types of legal restrictions on alcohol availability

Many governments provide for licensing of privately owned retail alcohol outlets. Regulations may govern the forms in which alcohol may be sold, the types of off-premises retail outlets permitted, the types of establishments for which on-premise licenses may be granted, and the hours of the day and days of the week during which alcohol may be sold by off- or on-premises outlets.

Public monopolies on off-premises retail sale of alcohol exist in some countries, such as Sweden, Norway, and Finland, and in some US states and Canadian provinces. Under a public monopoly, off-premises retail sale of alcohol is permitted only in state or local government stores. Public monopolies result in uniform retail prices for alcohol sold at off-premises establishments and fewer off-premises outlets at the local level.

Communities may regulate the locations and densities of alcohol outlets, through local powers to regulate and zone areas of a community for certain uses, or to place limits or restrictions on specific types of outlets. For example, communities may establish conditions for alcohol outlets as a part of their local business licenses. Such conditions may govern outlet types, locations (e.g., distances from schools, churches, or residential neighborhoods), and densities (e.g., number per geographic area or per unit of population). They also may specify requirements for lighting, accessibility to public transportation, server permits, minimum server age, and staff training in responsible hospitality (e.g., ensuring that servers are aware of the relevant laws or can recognize and not serve intoxicated persons). Communities may establish limits or bans on the use or sale of alcohol in public areas such as parks, beaches, stadiums, or arenas. (See discussion of such municipal policies in Canada by Douglas, 1990; and Gliksman et al., 1990, 1995.)

Formal regulation may address liability for harm resulting from licensee negligence in the service of alcohol. For example, a retailer may be liable for damage caused by intoxicated or underage patrons served by that establishment. This liability, often referred to as "dram-shop liability," is established either by legislation or by common-law precedent.

Social accessibility of alcohol may be controlled through restrictions on general accessibility (e.g., requirements that certain kinds of events be alcohol-free) or accessibility to youth (e.g., requirement of keg registration, to prevent beer from being made available to minors at a party). In some US states, common-law precedent exists for "social-host liability," to which a private person is exposed when serving alcohol in a social setting. Private individuals have been successfully sued for providing alcohol to minors or to intoxicated persons who subsequently were injured, or killed or harmed someone else. (For further discussion of liability issues, see Mosher, 1983; Wagenaar & Holder, 1991; and Holder et al., 1993.)

Governments may influence the economic availability of alcohol by taxing alcohol sales; alcohol is often an important source of government tax revenue. Governments also may regulate the retail prices of alcoholic beverages, by setting maximum, minimum, or fixed retail or wholesale prices, or by limiting price fluctuations.

Promotion and advertising of alcohol may be regulated through outright bans on alcohol advertising, or through restrictions on the types and forms of advertising or promotion (e.g., bans on billboard advertisements, point-of-purchase promotions, price promotions, or advertisement of alcohol prices). For example, Sweden, Finland, and Norway restrict alcohol advertising by forbidding advertising on television, and some communities in the US ban price promotions of alcohol at bars or restaurants, to prevent heavy consumption as a result of "happy hours" or offers of two drinks for the price of one.

Enforcement of formal regulations and controls

The Formal Regulation and Control Subsystem in the community enforces the laws and rules applying to local alcohol sales. The level of enforcement activity depends on the resources allocated to enforcement. Thus, the activities of alcohol control agencies may expand or contract in response to changes in the law and the resources available for action.

The existence of rules and the intensity of their enforcement reflect the community's social values. For example, although most industrialized countries set a minimum age for purchasing or consuming alcohol, the effective minimum age (the age at which a practical barrier to purchasing or consuming alcohol exists) depends on the level or intensity of enforcement of the minimum drinking age. If the law is not enforced, alcohol salespersons and servers will not be vigilant in checking proof of age, and underage persons will not be deterred from purchasing or consuming alcohol (see discussions and research by Wagenaar & Wolfson, 1994; Wolfson et al., 1996).

As interested and informed parties, producers of alcoholic beverages (who may or may not be located within the community system) play a role in the shaping of alcohol laws and regulations (Bunce et al., 1981). For example, they may attempt to influence the government to enact less-restrictive rules and regulations affecting wholesale and retail sales of alcohol. Furthermore, producers act in response to regulatory activities. For example, if laws specify the sale of 3.2 beer (3.2% alcohol by volume), the alcoholic beverage industry will be motivated to manufacture such beer (Brown & Wallace, 1980).

Figure 4.1 illustrates the basic structure of a Formal Regulation and Control Subsystem.

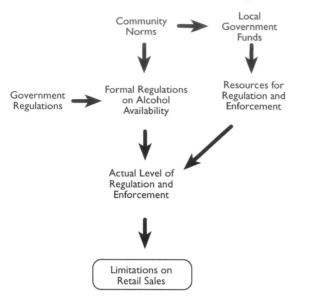

Figure 4.1 Formal Regulation and Control Subsystem.

Examples of government controls

Kortteinen (1989) has reviewed the formal regulations and controls of a number of industralized countries which have established some form of public retail monopoly for alcohol. In the US, formal controls on the sale and availability of alcoholic beverages have ranged from total prohibition under the 18th Amendment to the Constitution (1920–33) to a present trend toward liberalization. Control of alcoholic beverage sales has become primarily a state and local matter.[1] At the end of US Prohibition, state alcoholic beverage control (ABC) agencies were established in the states that legalized alcohol consumption. These agencies were given the mission of regulating the distribution of alcoholic beverages for the public good. The retail sale of alcohol in each state was regulated either through licensing of private retail stores or through establishment of state-operated monopoly retail stores. Regulatory practices in the "license" and "monopoly" states have since evolved.

1 Under the 21st Amendment to the Constitution and the Federal Alcohol Administration Act of 1935, the federal government maintains specific authorities in the areas of alcoholic beverage taxation, regulation of labeling and advertising, import controls, and control and enforcement pertaining to illicit alcohol production (Matlins, 1976, pp. 37–38).

In most countries, government control of alcohol sales covers the licensing of retail alcohol outlets by type of sale (on-premises or off-premises) and type of beverage (beer, wine, or spirits). In both types of alcohol control systems, on-premises alcohol outlets are owned and operated by private parties. In "license" situations, private retailers own and operate all off-sale premises outlets as well. In retail monopoly situations, the government controls the retail off-premises sales of alcohol. In a state monopoly, the government agency determines the number and location of off-premises retail outlets, hours of retail sales, and retail prices.

In licensing situations, the government controls privately owned outlets through the licensing process, which may restrict the types of businesses that can obtain licenses and may control the numbers, locations, and settings of private retail alcohol outlets. Location of outlets in what are considered to be in inappropriate community settings (for example, near churches or schools) may be prohibited, and the density of outlets in particular areas may be restricted. The government alcohol policy control specifies a ratio of alcohol outlets to persons. For example, in the US, California limits the number of bars, restaurants, and off-premises stores per unit population. Government regulations also can limit hours of sale, and can limit or prescribe serving and management practices. They can provide for dram-shop liability and requirements relating to lighting, availability of public transportation, staff age, staff drinking, and server training. For restaurants, the law can specify the percentage of sales that must be derived from food.

Government regulations can set maximum, minimum, or fixed prices for retail and wholesale alcohol sales, and can include measures that limit price fluctuations, such as requiring that the retail price listed for a specific brand of alcoholic beverage be no lower than the lowest price at which that product is sold to any wholesaler. Price posting may be required, whereby manufacturers and wholesalers must file schedules of case and bottle prices for their products with the government, and the prices must remain in effect for a specified time. Advertising and promotion, including price promotion, may be restricted or banned.

Government regulations can specify criminal penalties or administrative sanctions (e.g., fines, or license suspension or revocation) for violations by retail alcohol outlets, such as selling alcohol to minors, serving intoxicated persons, serving after hours, or serving without a license.

The powers given by the national (or state) government to local authorities vary considerably. Local law may allow communities to establish provisions that can place unique restrictions on alcohol outlets. Local governments may be permitted a role in the alcohol outlet licensing process. Local governments may have the authority to issue liquor licenses, approve or disapprove licenses, protest issuance of licenses, revoke or suspend licenses, or restrict licenses by means of zoning laws. They may be allowed to specify the types, numbers, and locations of outlets, and the hours and days when alcohol may be sold. Some US states give counties or municipalities the option to ban all sales of alcohol or to ban certain types of sales, such as sale of alcohol at gasoline stations, or at bars or restaurants. In Sweden, cities and municipalities can participate in discussions and decisions concerning alcohol licenses in their area. Opportunities for local regulation, control and/or influence about licensing exists in such countries as Australia and New Zealand.

If private licenses are permitted and the government receives a license application, the public may receive notice of license review (e.g., via mailings, newspaper advertisements, or signs at the proposed outlet location). The government agency may notify the local police department, attorney, and governing council. An investigation may be conducted and the government decides whether to issue the license. Decisions may be based on the following factors: proximity to schools, churches, hospitals, playgrounds, or residences, and how the outlet would affect them; concentration of outlets in the area (number per capita); crime rate in the area and whether the outlet would create or exacerbate a law-enforcement problem; character and record of the applicant; and local zoning ordinances. An investigator may hold up approval of the license until local zoning approval has been obtained. Citizens usually are allowed to participate in the licensing process. Some jurisdictions allow petitioning against issuance of new licenses and protests against renewal of licenses. The law may provide for public notices, hearings, grounds for protest, protest procedures, investigation procedures, and the appeals process. Protests can be made within a set time after an application for a new alcohol license or renewal for an existing license.

Community zoning may be used to grant two types of permits: regular permits, which are given on demand to business applicants who conform to the local planning and zoning code; and conditional use permits, which attach special conditions to the issuance of a business permit for a particular type of establishment. Regular permits can have text restrictions applying to certain types of retail stores and their locations and prohibiting certain operations. Examples of text restrictions include special security requirements, limitations on hours of operation, and required minimum distances between alcohol outlets and schools, churches, or residences, or between two alcohol outlets. Regular zoning permits are given automatically to individuals wishing to use property in ways allowed by zoning ordinances. However, for some kinds of property use, the law may require that conditional use permits be obtained. The zoning authorities can base the decision to grant a conditional use permit on already established criteria, or they may establish criteria at the time of review; thus, conditional use permits give local authorities considerable flexibility in controlling the use of property. Conditional use permits allow for local oversight of the operation of the outlet; if review standards are violated, the permit may be revoked, or the owner may be penalized.

The resources available to government agencies for carrying out their administrative, licensing, and enforcement activities vary. Low funding levels can hamper enforcement. Empirically, the level of enforcement in the US has been found to be related to the level or type of alcoholic beverage control; Gruenewald, Madden & Janes (1992) found that more resources are allocated for enforcement in monopoly states than in license states.

Interactions with other subsystems

The Formal Regulation and Control Subsystem is a complex adaptive system that adjusts to and influences other community subsystems. This subsystem acts as a gatekeeper, regulating the types and quantities of alcoholic beverages flowing into a specific jurisdiction, and placing limits on the physical and economic availability of alcoholic beverages to consumers within that jurisdiction.

The Social Norms Subsystem influences the creation of regulations. The legal regulations and restrictions established by a community reflect the concerns, desires, and values of the citizens. Thus, if alcohol is a socially undesired product, then total bans, prohibitions, or severe restrictions on alcohol's legal availability (as well as sanctions against illegal availability) will exist. If alcohol is a valued and socially desired product that is integrated into routine community life, then few restrictions may exist. Most communities fall between these extremes. Even where drinking is socially acceptable, if concern exists about dangers related to drinking, then restrictions intended to inhibit heavy or dangerous use of alcohol, or to reduce alcohol-involved problems, will be established. If drinking by young people is not desired, a minimum age for purchase or consumption of alcohol will exist.

Norms representing the community's values, preferences, and concerns about alcohol availability also are expressed through allocation of resources for enforcement. A community may have many formal restrictions, but little or no enforcement. On the other hand, a community may insist on full enforcement of rules and regulations, ensuring their effectiveness. Communities can influence enforcement by pressurizing enforcement agencies to be thorough and by providing sufficient resources to maintain full enforcement capacity.

The major output of the Formal Regulation and Control Subsystem is limits on the retail sale of alcohol in the community, which provide input to the Retail Sales Subsystem. The Retail Sales Subsystem provides input to the Consumption Subsystem, which in turn, through the Social, Economic, and Health Consequences Subsystem, influences all outcomes related to alcoholic beverage consumption, including alcohol-related accidents, morbidity and mortality, traffic deaths, social disruption, and reduced productivity at the workplace.

As an adaptive system, the Formal Regulation and Control Subsystem tends to maintain a balance between community norms and values, and the pressures of the retail alcohol market. If enforcement of restrictions on alcohol availability is severe, retailers may protest. If the level of enforcement is low, and alcohol-involved problems increase, citizens may protest.

The purpose of the Formal Regulation and Control Subsystem is to influence the form and extent of alcohol availability in the community. Does this work? Numerous studies have examined the relationships between regulation of alcohol availability, alcohol consumption, and alcohol-involved problems. The evidence consistently suggests that regulations and controls that restrict the availability of alcohol do reduce average per capita alcohol consumption and the rate of alcohol-involved problems (e.g., Rush & Gliksman, 1986). MacDonald & Whitehead (1983) noted that variation in the availability of alcohol accounts for some of the variance in alcohol consumption and in alcohol-involved problems. Gruenewald, Madden & Jones (1992) concluded that physical access to alcoholic beverages is related both to rates of alcohol consumption and to rates of alcohol-involved problems.

Thus, social values (expressed in the Social Norms Subsystem) influence legal regulation of the Retail Sales Subsystem, through pressure for restrictions and enforcement, and provision of the resources for enforcement. Enforcement of regulations through the Formal Regulation and Control Subsystem limits alcohol availability, which, in turn, limits alcohol consumption in the community. These subsystem interactions are illustrated in Fig. 4.2.

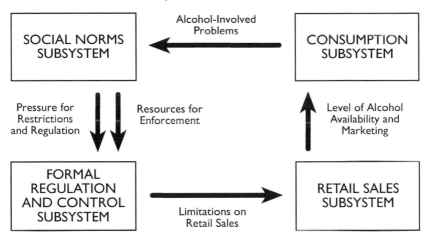

Figure 4.2 Interaction of Formal Regulation and Control Subsystem with Social Norms and Retail Sales Subsystems, and the link to Consumption Subsystem.

5

Social Norms Subsystem: community values and social influences that affect drinking

Introduction

The Social Norms Subsystem represents the social dynamics that influence rates and patterns of alcohol consumption in the community. The "norm" is a basic concept of social science, referring to informal social rules or proscriptions defining acceptable and unacceptable behavior within any social group, organization, or larger social structure, such as a village, small town, or city.

Norms are reflected in the homogeneity of behavior observable among any people with sufficient social contact and exposure. This homogeneity can exist even across entire societies with sufficient common exposure to language, social values, mass messages, and images. The US as a whole exhibits a notable homogeneity of values, despite regional differences in styles of behavior and values, as subgroups with their own common heritages (and languages) also are influenced by the larger social collectivity. For example, with respect to drinking norms, a three-generation study of Mexican-Americans (Markides, Krause & Mendes de Leon, 1988) showed that acculturation altered this ethnic group's traditional normative drinking patterns.

Drinking norms are social influences and pressures regarding acceptable drinking behavior, which may act either to encourage (permit) or to discourage (restrict) alcohol consumption. Drinking norms are part of a larger collection of norms influencing many types of individual and social behavior (see Pittman & Snyder, 1962; Pittman, 1967; Simpura, 1987; and Room, 1991). Community drinking norms reflect general attitudes about drinking and societal expectations regarding the levels of drinking considered appropriate. These expectations generally are expressed as a range of context-specific levels of acceptable alcohol consumption: what is considered appropriate drinking behavior depends on the location or occasion (e.g., at a bar, funeral, party, or at home). Drinking norms may also vary across demographic subgroups (e.g., by age, gender, religion, race, or ethnicity).

To apply the concept of cultural norms to drinking implies the existence of a set of informal social rules or guidelines for drinking that are recognized and shared by the collective (e.g., the community). Skog (1980, 1985) described this mechanism as social interaction in which any individual's drinking habits are strongly influenced by the drinking of friends and more generally by the drinking patterns of his or her social network. According to Skog (1985), drinking populations tend to act as collectives, their consumption levels increasing and decreasing in concert.

Reviewing international patterns of alcohol consumption in industrial societies, Holder & Janes (1989) argued that over the last two centuries, a number of industrialized countries have followed a regular pattern of consumption increases and decreases, creating cycles of consumption of roughly two generations, or 20 years. Room (1989) gave a cultural interpretation of these cycles, suggesting that generational responses to drinking produce alternating "wet" and "dry" periods.

This chapter first discusses how social norms influence alcohol consumption. It then describes measures used as indicators of drinking norms. Next, it discusses how various forces and factors influence drinking norms, acting through negative and positive feedback loops. The influence of community concern about drinking-related issues and social acceptability of drinking are explored in more detail. The chapter concludes with a summary of how the Social Norms Subsystem interacts with other subsystems.

The influence of social norms on alcohol consumption

Consumer behavior, like other behavior, is affected by cultural and societal values and norms. The values attached to possessions are not inherent in the possessions, but are assigned according to cultural factors. Markin (1974) argued that although income is a major determinant in consumer purchasing, consumer motivations, expectations, and aspirations also are major determinants of consumption. For example, the Kwakiutl Indians consider accumulation of goods to be undesirable, and they give goods away as part of community celebrations (Markin, 1974). Demand for goods is a function of their potential to solve problems, to make the consumer more socially acceptable, and to help the consumer attain a particular lifestyle or social position.

Thus, the desire to buy appears to be a function of consumer attitudes and expectations. Betancourt & Gautschi (1988) described consumer demand for a product as a function of retail price, quality, and retail service or availability, especially for commodities that yield satisfaction directly. Consumer demand for (or spending on) durable goods can be influenced by consumer confidence but spending on non-durable goods can be more influenced by consumer expectations. Partanen (1990) argued that alcohol is a symbol – a kind of language that can be used to express aspects of social life. He characterized alcohol as a medium of sociability, in that intoxication is conducive to a heightened sense of sociability and that drinking can be an act of social exchange involving fun, food, and social discourse. Consumers purchase goods like alcohol not only for their practical utility, but for their culturally determined symbolic significance.

Countries differ in alcohol consumption not only because of differences in the price and physical availability of alcohol, but also because of differences in social values and norms about drinking (Mäkelä et al., 1981). Examining time-series patterns of aggregate alcohol consumption in Norway, Skog (1986) concluded that economic development influenced consumption in both the 19th and 20th centuries. However, he also concluded that alcohol consumption cannot easily be predicted from economic development alone and that, to be more accurate, predictions should include social and cultural variables.

US per capita alcohol consumption from 1970 to 1994 also provides an example of how alcohol consumption cannot be accounted for simply by the economic factors of price and income. From 1970 to 1980, US per capita alcohol consumption rose steadily in accordance with increases in inflation-adjusted income and a decline in the price of alcohol relative to prices of other goods. However, after 1980, consumption began to decline, even though the relative price of alcohol continued to decline and adjusted income increased. By 1987, per capita consumption of alcohol had declined to the 1970 level, even though changes in price and income alone would have predicted a steady increase in consumption over the period. Treno, Parker & Holder (1993) conducted a multivariate time-series analysis to determine which factors most influenced per capita alcohol consumption in the US from 1950 to 1986. They found that personal income had a significant effect, but that price had only a slight influence when indicators of changes in social values and family activities were accounted for.

Gruenewald (1988) established four basic propositions concerning the relationship of social norms to alcohol consumption:

(1) Rates of alcohol consumption change over time, and current rates of alcohol use appear to be autocorrelated with previous levels of use.

(2) Social norms establish acceptable levels for the appearance of alcohol consumption in societies. Rates of consumption tend toward these "target" levels.

(3) Accessibility of alcohol constrains alcohol consumption in societies, through restraints both on alcohol availability and on the ability of consumers to purchase alcohol.

(4) Pure "demand" for alcohol is best represented by the target level of alcohol consumption in a society when constraints on accessibility are removed.

In an extensive empirical investigation of the relationship between drinking norms and actual alcohol consumption, Frankel & Whitehead (1981) examined evidence from 69 societies. They concluded that in societies where drinking customs, values, and sanctions are established, well known, and widely accepted, per capita consumption will be relatively low, and few persons in that society will consume in excess of 10 cl of absolute ethanol per day.

Types of drinking norms and their influence on alcohol-involved problems

In an international study involving cross-cultural comparisons of drinking and alcohol-involved problems, Österberg (1991) noted that the nature of the alcohol-involved problems found in each society varies according to the societies' specific social circumstances and drinking habits. Bales (1946) asserted that cultures or social structures can influence the rate of heavy drinking (and thus alcoholism) in three ways:

(1) According to the "stress hypothesis," sociostructural factors create stress and inner tension for members of society or of a subgroup.

(2) According to the "normative hypothesis," the culture defines whether drinking and intoxication can be used acceptably as a means to relieve stress and tension.

(3) According to the "functional alternative hypothesis," the cultural or social structure may or may not provide alternatives to alcohol for relief of stress and tension.

Bales explained the high rates of heavy drinking among men in 19th- and early-20th-century Ireland as the result of tension and frustration produced by a social structure that denied young men the opportunity for either sexual or status fulfillment. Concurrently, drinking norms permitted and even encouraged heavy drinking in local taverns as a way of dealing with personal stress. Following Bales, Pittman (1967) classified drinking norms into four categories: abstinent, ambivalent, permissive, and overpermissive.

Larsen & Abu-Laban (1968) examined the relationship between three types of drinking norms and drinking that deviates from these norms:

(1) "Proscriptive" norms prohibit any drinking; any drinking is considered deviant.
(2) "Prescriptive" norms sanction drinking, but with established limits on the appropriate consumption level for any occasion; heavy drinking is considered deviant. For example, prescriptive norms might define the following drinking patterns and levels as deviant: drinking alcohol at least once a month or more often and consuming four or more drinks in a sitting, or drinking twice a week or more and consuming three or more drinks in a sitting.
(3) "Non-scriptive" norms neither prohibit drinking nor provide adequate guidelines for drinking behavior. They incompletely specify acceptable drinking behavior and the generality of drinking standards.

Proscriptive and non-scriptive norms are alike in providing little guidance on drinking behavior, but they differ in that proscriptive norms forbid drinking, while non-scriptive norms do not. Prescriptive and non-scriptive norms are alike in permitting drinking, but non-scriptive norms give little or no guidance on drinking behavior, while prescriptive norms can provide elaborate sets of guidelines.

Larsen & Abu-Laban (1968) found that the heaviest drinking occurs in social environments governed by non-scriptive norms; less drinking occurs in environments with prescriptive norms, and drinking levels are lowest under proscriptive norms. Most significantly, they found that the strength of the norm depends on the importance of the norm's source to the individual. That is, whether or not a person abides by the norms of the group depends on the degree to which the group has meaning or relevance for that individual.

Linsky, Straus & Colby (1985) undertook a test of Bales's 1946 theory concerning culturally supported attitudes towards drinking and intoxication, using US data at the state level. They found that both high community rates of stressful life events (such as divorce or loss of work) and indicators of stressful conditions (such as poor community economic conditions, low welfare status, and low live birth rates) are correlated with indicators of heavy alcohol consumption. In a follow-up study, Linsky, Colby & Straus (1986) found that the existence of proscriptive norms is negatively correlated with heavy drinking but positively correlated with indicators of social disruptiveness of alcohol use (such as alcohol-involved arrests).

Indicators of drinking norms

The socially acceptable (i.e., normative) level of drinking is assumed to be indicated by the actual aggregate drinking level. However, drinking surveys, which might appear to be the best indicator of the aggregate drinking level, consistently account for only 50% or less of alcohol sales in most countries. For this reason, researchers have typically used retail sales of all alcoholic beverages per capita as an apparent indicator of aggregate consumption (e.g., Loeb, 1978; Cook & Tauchen, 1982, 1984; Hoadley, Fuchs & Holder, 1984; Kendell, 1984). The question remains of how to relate the aggregate consumption distribution to socially acceptable consumption. At least three alternative measures might be used to define the norm:

(1) A measure of central tendency (i.e., an average).
(2) An upper limit for consumption.
(3) An acceptable range of consumption.

Measures of central tendency. The aggregate drinking norm may be defined as the average (mean, median, or modal) consumption level. Population consumption is most frequently represented by the mean (numeric average) per capita consumption. However, the mean is strongly influenced by values at the extremes of the distribution; it well represents the normative consumption level only if the consumption distribution is bell-shaped. The median and mode are less influenced by extreme values. The median consumption level (i.e., the half-way point in the distribution) divides the drinking population into two equal parts. The mode is the most common consumption level (i.e., the level that represents the largest number of people), assuming that the consumption distribution is unimodal. If the distribution is bell-shaped, then the median, mode, and mean are identical or very close in value. As discussed in Chapter 2, the actual distribution of alcohol consumption in most cultures is not bell-shaped, but is skewed towards the right (see Fig. 2.1 in Chapter 2). In this distribution, the long tail extending to the right represents individuals who drink far in excess of typical levels, and are likely to be judged as deviant and possibly dependent upon alcohol.

Using drinking survey data and alcohol sales data from a number of countries, Skog (1985) demonstrated empirically that levels of national mean absolute alcohol consumption could be used to make reasonable estimates of the distribution of drinkers among consumption categories. Skog further argued that as mean consumption increases, the rate of increase in consumption differs across consumption groups; for example, a 1% increase in mean consumption would be expected to correspond to a larger rate of increase in consumption among light and medium drinkers than among heavy drinkers.

At the local or community level, use of mean per capita alcohol sales as an indicator of social drinking norms has the following disadvantages:

(1) Local sales include purchases by non-residents (such as tourists or commuters).
(2) For many locations, such as US states, sales data are based on shipments to wholesalers. Depending on the territories of individual wholesalers, shipment data may not reflect all wholesale shipments to a specific community, city, or county.
(3) Sales are a measure of purchases and not of immediate consumption. For example, delays in consumption result when wine is stored for aging or when an open bottle of spirits is served from over time.

Upper limit on consumption. An alternative approach is to define the aggregate drinking norm with respect to an upper limit on consumption. This level is considered to be the upper bound for socially acceptable drinking over a given period or per drinking occasion; all drinking below this level is accepted as normative. The use of an upper limit is based on the assumption that all lower levels of drinking, including abstinence, are socially acceptable. Figure 5.1 illustrates the use of an upper limit to define a drinking norm; all drinking above this level would be considered socially deviant.

Acceptable range of consumption. A third alternative is to define the drinking norm as a range of acceptable consumption levels, with lower and upper bounds. From this perspective, drinking at either higher or lower levels is viewed as deviant, and social pressure exists for consuming less than the amount of alcohol that defines the higher bound of the acceptable range and more than the lower bound of the acceptable range. This approach is illustrated in Fig. 5.2. In a society or subgroup where alcohol has a prominent and socially important role, drinking will be normative, and abstinence will be socially discouraged. This appears to be the situ-

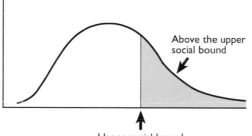

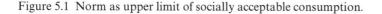

Figure 5.1 Norm as upper limit of socially acceptable consumption.

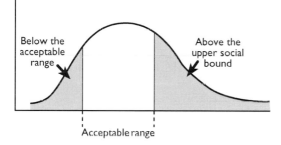

Figure 5.2 Norm as a range of socially acceptable consumption.

ation in most social groups, e.g., among the subgroup of males between 18 and 25 years old, drinking is a major activity and expected of all sub-group members, therefore, a high level of consumption per occasion is normative.

Negative and positive pressures on drinking norms

Within the community system, drinking norms are subjected to both positive pressures (favoring increased drinking) and negative pressures (favoring decreased drinking). When the positive and negative pressures are balanced, the norm for alcohol consumption oscillates around an equilibrium level. This stable state is illustrated in the top part of Fig. 5.3. If positive pressures dominate, the drinking norm shifts upwards. For example, if actual per capita consumption increases while all other factors (e.g., the price of alcohol) remain unchanged, then positive pressures are dominant, and the socially acceptable level of drinking (i.e., the norm)

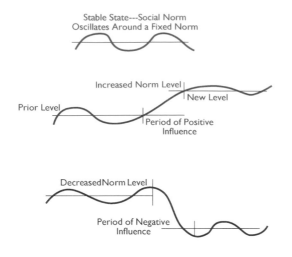

Figure 5.3 Illustration of stable, increased, and decreased norm levels about drinking.

increases, at least until negative pressures again balance positive pressures. This shift to an increased normative consumption level is illustrated in the middle part of Fig. 5.3. If the actual level of consumption decreases while all other factors remain equal, then negative factors are dominant, and the norm decreases, as shown in the bottom part of Fig. 5.3. (For discussion of the dynamics, development, and maintenance of norms and values within a social system, see Axelrod, 1986; and Epstein & Axtell, 1996.)

At the individual level, drinking norms can be conceptualized as establishing acceptable levels for personal drinking. A number of potential inhibitors or barriers to drinking are socially established. For example, drinking may be illegal (e.g., for persons under 18 or 21 years of age). Drinking may be considered immoral and thus be blocked by proscriptions forbidding drinking or limiting the amount of alcohol consumed. Drinking may be viewed as dangerous to personal health or safety (e.g., through its role in automobile crashes). Drinking may be seen as non-functional, or disruptive to acceptable or desired social interaction or performance (e.g., at work or with one's family). Alcohol's ability to alter reality may be considered undesirable (for example, a recovering alcoholic or a life-long abstainer may believe that "reality is better"). Each of these barriers works to establish the individual's personal norm for alcohol use in general or for the appropriate consumption levels in specific contexts (such as before or while driving).

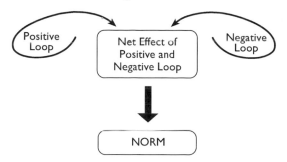

Figure 5.4 Norms about drinking as the result of positive and negative loops.

Generalizing to the community at large, both the attractiveness of alcohol use and the barriers to drinking have their effects at the group level. Overall societal drinking norms can be viewed as a function of three broad types of factors:

(1) General societal attitudes towards the use of alcohol. For example, such attitudes may be reflected in the display of alcohol in advertising or the mass media.
(2) Situation-specific norms. Examples include prohibitions against drinking at fraternity parties, and against drinking and driving. Norms against drinking and driving have been quite salient in the US over the past 10 to 15 years, and have strongly influenced overall drinking norms.
(3) Variations in drinking norms across subgroups. Expectations for drinking behavior vary with age and ethnic group, as well as with changes in the population mix. Although the gender mix itself is reasonably stable, drinking norms for women appear to have changed in many cultures, thus influencing the overall drinking norms.

Figure 5.4 illustrates how drinking norms (defined in terms of acceptable levels) are influenced by both positive (amplifying) and negative (dampening) feedback loops.

The negative loop reflects pressures that tend to limit the level of drinking considered socially acceptable – in particular, the importance of proscriptive norms and the level of public concern regarding the negative consequences of alcohol use. Some consequences of alcohol use are, at some level and under some conditions, perceived by society as negative. The level of these consequences and the level of public concern about them determine, at least indirectly, the socially acceptable level of consumption.

Perceived increases in problems such as drinking and driving crashes, violence related to drinking, alcohol-involved injuries and deaths, drinking by youths, or public disruption (public drunkenness, noise, or rowdiness involving drinking, trash, or concurrent drug sales) can increase social concern, as discussed in Chapter 7. As public concern about consumption rises, the level of consumption considered to be socially acceptable declines. However, there could be a lag between changes in the actual level of consumption in response to changes in norms.

The positive loop reflects pressures that interact to shift drinking norms to a new, higher level. For example, the social desirability of drinking may be enhanced by current levels of drinking and other influences, such as retail promotion of alcohol and mass-media portrayals of drinking. To the extent that drinking behavior is widespread or perceived to be widespread, it leads to increased social acceptance of drinking, which in turn maintains or increases socially acceptable drinking levels. For instance, if the actual drinking level is relatively constant, the existing beliefs and attitudes of members of society are reinforced at that level. This process also serves to socialize new members of society. When there is a time lag in the public recognition of a change in drinking levels, social desirability of drinking at any given time may be more strongly related to actual drinking in the recent past than to current drinking levels.

Specific influences that contribute to the positive and negative loops are illustrated in Fig. 5.5.

Community concern about alcohol use

The negative feedback loop represents the process by which community concern about alcohol use interacts with consumption levels to maintain stable drinking norms. Concern generally reflects awareness, or even fear, of the negative consequences of drinking. For concern to remain at a constant level, public awareness of specific alcohol-involved problems must be maintained or reinforced. Public awareness of alcohol-involved problems depends on the public's exposure to problems, which in most industrialized communities occurs via the mass media, through news or feature coverage of problems associated with drinking, or through purposeful public education and awareness campaigns. Without reinforcement, concern gradually decays (i.e., decreases to zero) over time. Thus, the level of concern about alcohol use in a community is the product of two opposing forces: increases in public awareness of alcohol-involved problems, and the natural decay of concern if it is not reinforced.

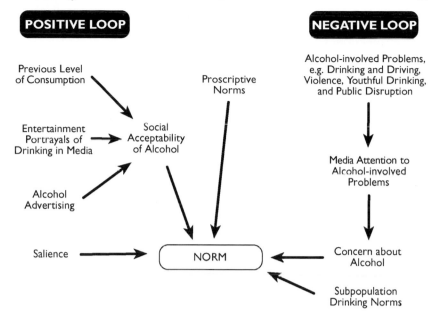

Figure 5.5 Possible factors contributing to positive and negative loops influencing social norms about drinking.

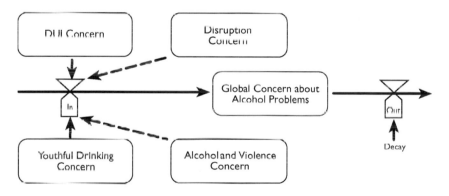

Figure 5.6 Community concern about alcohol problems.

The dynamics of community concern about alcohol use are illustrated in Fig. 5.6. Specific concerns about alcohol use (e.g., driving under influence (DUI) of alcohol, drinking by youths, public disruption, and violence) are combined as inputs to global concern about alcohol-involved problems in the community. (The influences of these specific concerns are not necessar-

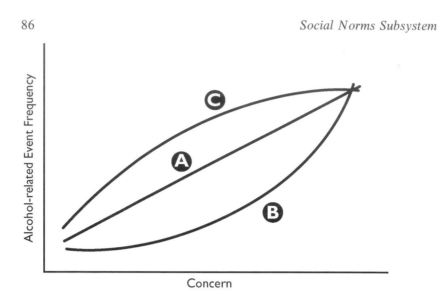

Figure 5.7 Direct relationship of problem frequency to concern.

ily additive or of equal importance.) Without new input, the level of global concern spontaneously decays.

The negative feedback loop may be conceptualized in several ways, depending on how concern is defined. The simplest approach is to assume that the level of community concern about an alcohol-involved event is simply a function of the observed frequency of the event. In this approach, an alcohol-involved problem is, by definition, any event or outcome that can distress or upset others (e.g., admissions for alcoholism, traffic crash deaths, public drinking, noise connected to drinking, or alcohol-involved violence). Figure 5.7 illustrates possible relationships between event frequency (the observed number of events) and level of concern. Curve A is a linear relationship – a unit increase in the frequency of an event produces a corresponding unit increase in concern. Curves B and C illustrate non-linear relationships between event frequency and concern – as event frequency increases, curve B shows concern accelerating, and curve C shows concern leveling off after a certain point.

A more complex approach defines concern as related not only to the frequency of an alcohol-involved event, but also to the locally assigned or perceived significance of the event to the community. Significance refers to the degree to which a community feels or perceives that an alcohol-involved event requires community response. The level of community concern is a function of both alcohol-involved event frequency and assigned significance. An alcohol-involved event is not a "problem" *per se*; it

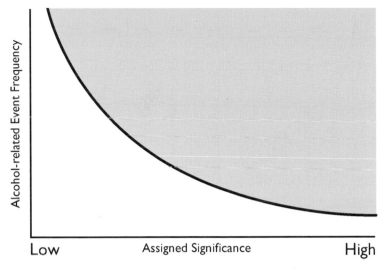

Figure 5.8 Concern as the interrelationship of problem frequency and significance to the community.

becomes a problem when the significance assigned to that event by the community reaches a certain level, and the community becomes concerned about it. Thus, a threshold exists for community concern about an alcohol-involved event (i.e., whether or not it is considered to be a problem).

Figure 5.8 illustrates one way in which community concern may be expressed as a function of event frequency and assigned significance. The line represents the threshold for concern, and the shaded area above represents the domain of concern. If significance is low, then even if the event frequency is high, the community may be largely unconcerned. For example, public drunkenness in inner cities frequently is tolerated even when it is common. On the other hand, if significance is high, then even relatively infrequent events can cause concern. For example, the frequency of birth defects among live births resulting from heavy drinking during pregnancy is low. However, the significance of birth defects to the community has been great enough in some instances to result in local requirements for warning labels about drinking during pregnancy.

Alternatively, concern may be expressed as a series (family) of curves, each representing a discrete level of concern. Within this family of curves, each level of concern may be achieved through various combinations of event frequency and assigned significance. For example, Fig. 5.9 shows curves for alcohol-involved events where concern is low (A), mild (B), medium (C), or high (D).

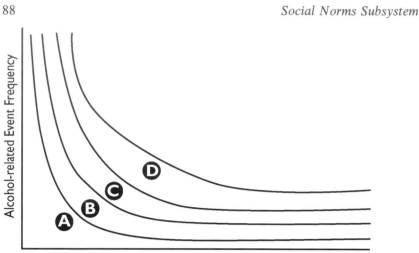

Assigned Significance

Figure 5.9 Illustration of a family of community concern curves.

Examples of international efforts to purposefully increase community concern about heavy drinking include a community-based public education campaign in New Zealand (Casswell & Gilmore, 1989; Casswell et al., 1989), a French campaign to portray the negative effect of intoxication (Comiti, 1990), and Canadian mass-media campaigns to increase public concern about drinking in recreational areas and support for policies restricting such drinking (Gliksman, 1986; Gliksman et al., 1990; Douglas, 1990).

Social acceptability of drinking

The positive feedback loop reflects the social acceptability of drinking, which is a function of its attractiveness and social desirability. All other things being equal, alcohol's social acceptability and actual consumption level change in the same direction, and reinforce each other: an increase in consumption results in increased acceptability, and increased acceptability results in increased consumption.

This positive feedback relationship between acceptability and consumption could involve a threshold effect, such that acceptability changes only in response to consumption changes above a specified magnitude. In this type of relationship, the change in acceptability could be defined as proportional to the change in consumption. Therefore, a threshold effect is unlikely to make much difference unless it is quite large. In such a case, a change in consumption large enough to exceed the threshold would result in an abrupt, large change in social acceptability. However, in the US, large changes per capita alcohol consumption do not occur over a short period (such as a year). From 1970 to 1990, the largest annual change in per capita consumption of absolute ethanol in the US was an increase of only 2.8% between 1970 and 1971, a percentage change unlikely in itself to produce a dynamic change in social acceptability. Thus, it appears more likely that the relationship could be a simple incremental one.

The extent of drinking shown in the mass media (e.g., in advertising and television shows) is probably an important factor reinforcing social desirability of alcohol consumption. However, the dynamics of such an effect are complex. For example, media portrayals of alcohol use may affect drinking norms, but they can also be viewed as a measure or function of the norms.

The effect of advertising on alcohol consumption has been a source of considerable debate (Smart, 1988; Saffer, 1993). The ability of advertising to increase other substance use (e.g., cigarette smoking) has been demonstrated (see Klitzner, Gruenewald & Bamberger, 1991). With respect to alcohol, investigators have disagreed as to whether the empirical evidence shows that advertising directly stimulates consumption (i.e., an increase in advertising causes an immediate increase in consumption). Alternatively, advertising may affect consumption through delayed social reinforcement. This view suggests that alcohol advertising has two functions: immediate stimulus or reinforcement of brand preference; and long-term (delayed) reinforcement of the social attractiveness or desirability of drinking in general. Empirical evidence of this reinforcement potential has been reported by Grube & Wallack (1994), who found that pre-adolescent exposure to alcohol advertising is causally linked to expressed intent to drink in the future.

Another influence on the perceived social desirability of alcohol is the portrayal of drinking in entertainment (e.g., in television shows). Media portrayals of drinking contribute to individuals' perceptions of its pervasiveness. In the US, the portrayal of drinking in prime time television shows, while declining over the 1980s could serve to socially reinforce a conclusion that "drinking is popular" or "undertaken by everyone." Drinking in such television shows occurs more frequently than drinking occurs in real life and alcohol is shown as being consumed much more often than water. (See Wallack et al., 1990.)

The more pervasive consumption is in a community, the greater its effect on individuals' consumption (Skog, 1985). To the extent, therefore, that a

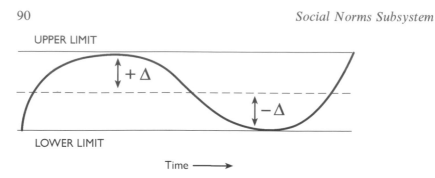

Figure 5.10 salience oscillating around a specific value over time.

community's per capita consumption exceeds or falls below the national average, the effects of media exposure on the social acceptability of alcohol may have greater or lesser effects on consumption.

The concept of salience

In the Social Norms Subsystem, the value of the community norm for alcohol consumption at any point in time is defined as the net result of positive and negative forces. "Salience" is an intervening variable that can enhance the effects of these negative and positive forces on the norm. Salience reflects the importance of drinking-related issues in people's lives at a given time. The concept of salience is based on observed changes in the importance of drinking-related issues in most industrialized countries from the 1970s to the 1980s. In the US, public attention to drinking-related issues in the 1980s was associated with later real declines in per capita consumption. Not only did concern about alcohol-involved problems become more influential, but the relative importance of drinking in people's lives changed. This relative importance is expressed in the Social Norms Subsystem by the factor of salience.

Salience may be considered to function as a dynamic elasticity in the strength of a positive or negative influence on the norm. As an explanatory variable, salience may be defined as varying within a set range over time unless stimulated to reach a new level. Figure 5.10 shows salience oscillating around a specific salience value, within upper (represented by $+ \Delta$ or higher than the current salience) and lower (represented by $- \Delta$) limits.

External pressure (a shock to the system) can cause salience to move outside of its existing range. Salience may increase in response to threat or fear related to alcohol use, or in response to pleasure and social desirability

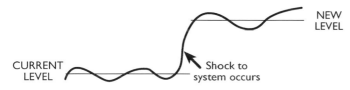

Figure 5.11 Salience seeks new level.

of drinking. For example, Fig. 5.11 illustrates the case where a new stimulus increases personal attention to drinking (for example, via personal or group experience with a drinking and driving crash, or via media attention to potential health benefits of drinking wine). In such a case, salience may break out of its stable range and reach a new level. As shown in Fig. 5.11, salience then oscillates around a new, higher stable level. It may be argued that in the early 1980s in the US, increased national news coverage of drinking and driving in the US provided a shock that increased the salience of drinking-related issues. In other words, the news coverage caused a step transformation that pushed salience through a threshold to a new level. Empirical evidence of increased attention to alcohol in the US is provided by national surveys (Clark & Hilton, 1991), as well as measures of media attention to alcohol-involved problems (Mouden & Russell 1994).

Once salience reaches a new level, three outcomes are possible:

(1) This new level may be self-maintaining (i.e., salience may oscillate around the new level).
(2) A shock may occur that further increases salience.
(3) Salience may decay over time, reaching some lower stable level.

Salience may be maintained by social reinforcement, as discussions about drinking-related issues become a part of routine life. On the other hand, as the pressures and attention that raised salience to a new level disappear, weaken, or become incorporated into routine life, salience may gradually decay.

Subgroup drinking norms

Important subpopulations in a community (subgroups based on age, gender, religion, ethnicity, or race) may have their own specific drinking norms, which may change independently over time, as illustrated in Fig. 5.12. The overall community drinking norm may be conceptualized as the mean (or unweighted average) of the norms for all important subgroups,

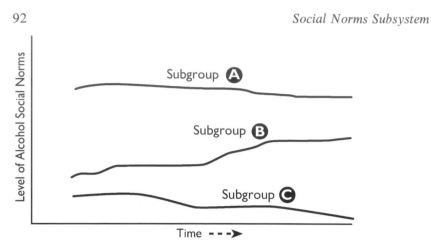

Figure 5.12 Social norms about drinking over time in different subgroups.

where each subgroup contributes to the total by its relative size or some other relative weight, such as its social influence in the community.

National surveys have shown that ethnic subgroups have specific drinking norms, which may differ significantly from the national norm (Clark & Midanik, 1982; Hilton, 1988). For example, the aggregate drinking levels for African-Americans in the US are lower than the overall national levels for both genders (Herd, 1991). Mexican-American women tend to drink far less than the norm for American women as a whole, whereas Mexican-American men have about the same average consumption level as American men as a whole, although their drinking patterns differ (Caetano, 1987, 1991).

According to Skog (1980), a change in overall per capita consumption does not necessarily entail identical changes in all subgroups with respect to alcohol consumption levels or the prevalence of heavy drinkers. In some instances, changes initially affect only specific subgroups. However, as Skog (1980) points out, if people in the affected subgroups interact with members of other subgroups, the change may eventually spread to these other subgroups. Such effects depend on the degree of interconnectedness between the subgroups. Isolated subgroups may change their drinking levels and patterns in a relatively independent manner. Thus, the rate at which changes in drinking behavior and norms diffuse among subgroups will depend on the structure of the community, and the location of the initial change in consumption.

Skog (1980) observed that the heterogeneity of consumption within a society (the extent to which different subgroups have different consumption levels) depends on two factors: the extent to which factors, such as price of alcohol relative to income and existing drinking norms, prescribe different consumption levels for different subgroups; and the extent to which members of different subgroups interact. Changes in the interconnectedness of subgroups – caused, for example, by increased physical mobility, or by increased or decreased social mobility – can result in changes in the heterogeneity of consumption levels or the prevalence of heavy drinkers among subgroups.

One perspective on subgroup norms comes from social control theory, which describes the origin and maintenance of norms, and their relation to sanctions (Hirschi, 1969; Meier, 1982). "Social control" has been defined as a process that links individuals with one another and with larger social structures. In social control theory, deviant behavior is defined as independent action by subgroups or individuals. The relative importance of social bonds can vary across racial or ethnic groups as a result of different emphases in the socialization process. For example, family structure may affect the elements of the social bond differently across racial groups. The degree to which an individual deviates from the aggregate norm depends on how well attached that person is to the overall community.

An alternative perspective on conformity and deviance comes from differential association theory. Sutherland (1947) noted that modern industrial societies incorporate multiple – often conflicting – norms, behavior patterns, and definitions of appropriate behavior. He posited that normative conflict is reflected in the existence of groups defined by their rates of deviant behavior (such as delinquency). For example, the extent to which a group is organized for or against delinquency determines its rate of law violation or crime, and the existence of groups defined by different crime rates reflects the existence of conflicting norms within the society.

One distinguishing characteristic of differential association theory is that it defines "deviance" not by acts, but by the relationship of acts to norms. Each person acts in accordance with his or her perception of cultural and social norms. However, norms differ from one subculture to another, and the norms of some subcultures will be considered deviant by society at large. An individual may commit a "deviant" act for two reasons: the individual is following the norms of his or her own subculture, which is considered deviant by the larger community; or the individual may be poorly integrated into a subculture not defined as deviant. In two separate analyses, Matsueda (1982) and Matsueda & Heimer (1987) concluded that differential association theory better explains the development of delinquency in both white and black populations than does the social control theory advanced by Hirschi (1969).

According to differential association theory, then, subgroups within a community may have diverse norms for drinking, and different acceptable drinking levels may exist within the context of an overall community norm. The work of Rabow & Watts (1982) and Donnelly (1978) support the notion that differential subgroup drinking levels are based (in part) on differential norms concerning drinking. Furthermore, subgroup differences in alcohol-related parameters, such as drinking and driving behavior, cirrhosis rates, or relative alcohol availability, can influence overall community norms about drinking, as members of different subgroups interact.

Interaction with other subsystems

The Social Norms Subsystem is continually adjusting to the pressures of positive and negative forces, through the feedback loops described in this chapter. These feedback loops are themselves influenced by factors outside the subsystem, including actual alcohol consumption and the frequency of alcohol-involved problems.

The Social Norms Subsystem is influenced by the Social, Economic, and Health Consequences Subsystem, since the extent of alcohol-involved problems can affect levels of community concern about alcohol-related issues. In turn, the Social Norms Subsystem influences the Legal Sanctions Subsystem and the Formal Regulation and Control Subsystem. Community concern about specific alcohol-involved problems (such as drinking and driving or drinking by underage persons) not only contributes to the overall level of community concern about drinking, but also influences enforcement activities in these other subsystems. As shown in Fig. 5.13, concern about drinking and driving can influence the level of enforcement of drinking under the influence of alcohol (DUI) laws, and concern about drinking by youths can influence the enforcement of laws against retail sale of alcohol to underage persons.

The Social Norms and Consumption Subsystems also interact in a feedback relationship. It may be assumed that the influence of drinking norms on actual alcohol consumption depends on the size of the difference between the socially acceptable and actual levels of consumption. When the acceptable level is lower than actual consumption, norms can discourage consumption. Conversely, when the acceptable level exceeds actual consumption, norms can stimulate consumption.

Figure 5.14 illustrates the expected interaction between normative and actual per capita consumption, as used in *SimCom*. The normative level is the average of the maximum acceptable levels of consumption from the

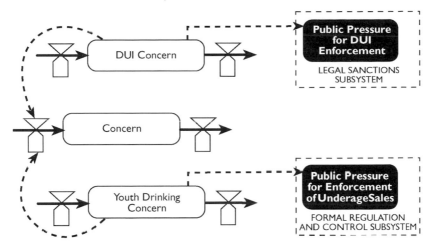

Figure 5.13 Illustration of specific community concerns within the Social Norms Subsystem can influence the Legal Sanctions and the Formal Regulation and Control subsystems.

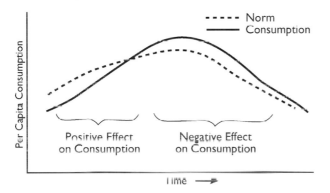

Figure 5.14 Illustration of the interaction of norm and consumption over time.

web of social networks that make up a given community (following Skog, 1985). The first part of the time-series curve shows that the normative consumption level exceeds actual consumption, so consumption increases towards the socially acceptable level. As some drinkers alter their consumption to this higher limit, a "spread of effect" occurs (Skog, 1985), whereby all drinkers proportionally adjust their consumption upward. At some point, actual consumption exceeds the normative level. With increasing concern about drinking and its consequences, the normative level starts to decrease. At this point, the pressure of social norms begins to draw consumption downwards, as drinkers seek to maintain their consumption within acceptable social limits. The wider the gap between the normative and actual consumption levels, the greater the pressure to bring consumption into line. This pressure is assumed to be non-linear (as discussed in Chapter 2).

6

Legal Sanctions Subsystem: prohibited uses of alcohol

Introduction

The Legal Sanctions Subsystem reflects the community's use of police powers to respond to and control alcohol-involved behaviors and events that are defined as illegal. Along with the Formal Control and Regulation Subsystem, the Legal Sanctions Subsystem is also involved in detecting and punishing those who violate specific rules concerning the possession and use of alcohol. The purpose of enforcement is not only to punish those who violate the laws or rules, but also to deter or prevent such behaviors or events through the threat of punishment.

Behaviors and events subject to enforcement within the Legal Sanctions Subsystem can include public intoxication or public drinking, alcohol-involved violent behavior, illegal sale of alcoholic beverages, drinking in places where it is prohibited (such as parks or beaches), and driving under the influence of alcohol (DUI). This chapter first briefly summarizes enforcement considerations in each of these areas. The rest of the chapter focuses primarily on drinking and driving, which is the dominant concern of this subsystem in many industrialized communities. The discussion of drinking and driving provides a detailed example of how the Legal Sanctions Subsystem functions and interacts with other subsystems in all aspects of enforcement.

Areas of enforcement within the subsystem

A common function of the Legal Sanctions Subsystem is detection and deterrence of public intoxication. Even where alcohol sales and consumption are legal, many communities in industrialized countries have defined intoxication in public view as illegal. As a result, the offense of public intoxication can consume considerable police time and court resources.

"Revolving-door drunks" are persons who, inebriated daily, are routinely arrested, jailed, taken to court for sentencing, and then returned to the street, only to become inebriated again and be re-arrested. Where the community's aversion to public intoxication is great, local police may have the task of clearing the streets of public drunks every day. For example, in downtown Atlanta, Georgia, in the 1970s, over 60% of patrol officer time was consumed by picking up and detaining public drunks (Cook et al., 1973). Although public intoxication remains illegal in many US and European communities, the trend has been for communities to develop alternatives to law-enforcement responses to this problem (as discussed in Chapter 7).

Alcohol-involved crime, both violent and non-violent, is the domain of local law enforcement. In the US, interviews with incarcerated offenders indicate that nearly 50% of them had been drinking when they committed the crime (Parker & Rebhun, 1995). While it is difficult to determine the causal role of alcohol in the committing of crimes, it is easier to understand how drinking contributes to the risk of victimization by reducing awareness and caution, and placing individuals at risk of assault (see Parker & Rebhun, 1995). A common function of the Legal Sanctions Subsystem is to respond to fights and assaults in which one or more of the participants has been drinking. In some communities, pub or bar fights are commonplace and considered a routine behavior associated with drinking. In other communities, alcohol-involved violent behavior is not tolerated, and law enforcement is used to deter or intervene in such behavior.

Where retail sale of alcohol in general or to certain groups is illegal, law enforcement is assigned the task of preventing such sale. For some time in the 19th and early 20th centuries, sale of alcohol to American Indians and other racial minorities in the US was banned, and the bans were enforced by police power. More recently, the primary group banned from purchasing alcohol (and, in some locations, from drinking at all) are persons under a certain age. By 1989, all states in the US established a minimum purchase (or drinking) age of 21 years for all types of alcoholic beverages. Before this time, the minimum age for alcohol varied among states and among types of alcoholic beverages, ranging from 18 for all beverages to 21 for all beverages and including other combinations (e.g., 18 for beer and wine, and 21 for spirits). Although the minimum age for purchase of alcohol in the US is defined at the state level, the degree of enforcement (and thus compliance) varies across communities. The Legal Sanctions Subsystem, along with the Formal Regulation and Control Subsystem, responds to social pressure by enforcing the minimum age for purchase or drinking of alcohol. Local law enforcement also has the responsibility for enforcing local bans on drinking in certain locations, such as public beaches, parks, or sports stadiums.

"Drinking and driving" refers to the tendency of the population to drive at various levels of intoxication or impairment. Drinking and driving behavior reflects the complex interplay of various demographic, economic, and social factors. In industrialized communities with large driving populations, enforcement of laws against drinking and driving can be a dominant function of the Legal Sanctions Subsystem. Traffic accidents involving alcohol are a major problem in most developed countries. In the US, fatal traffic crashes are the leading cause of death for persons under 40, translating into approximately one death every 11 minutes, and alcohol is a contributing factor in as many as 50% of these deaths (Zobeck et al., 1991). Not all cultures experience or identify drinking and driving as a major problem. However, drinking and driving is discussed in detail here to illustrate how the Legal Sanctions Subsystem functions.

Distribution of driving events as a function of blood alcohol concentration

Drinking and driving events are related to community drinking patterns: the more alcohol is a routine part of daily life, the more likely people will be to drive after (or while) drinking, all things being equal. Within any alcohol consumption class (as defined in Chapter 2), the number of drinking and driving events per capita reflects the frequency and quantity of alcohol consumption of that consumption class. As one moves from lower to higher consumption classes, the number of alcohol-involved driving events per person increases. For example, consumption class 1 has, on average, many fewer drinking and driving events per person than consumption class 4.

The amount of alcohol absorbed into the blood depends not only on the amount of alcohol consumed, but on body weight, concurrent consumption of food, and the rate at which alcohol is consumed. The more alcohol is absorbed into the blood, the greater the impairment of cognitive and physical skills, and the more impaired a person is in carrying out the demanding tasks of driving. The chief indicator of impairment is the blood alcohol concentration (BAC). The degree of impairment at a given BAC depends in part on the individual's drinking experience. However, on average, the higher the BAC, the greater the impairment.

Driving events can be distributed by the BACs of the drivers. The general distribution of drinking and driving is illustrated in Fig. 6.1, which shows the probability of a driving event as a function of BAC (for the population

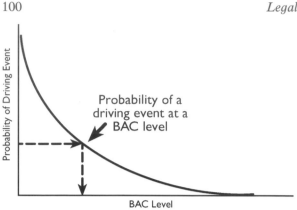

Figure 6.1 Description of possible functional form for driving event to BAC relationship.

as a whole). The most likely driving events are those at or near BAC = 0.0%. As the BAC of the driver increases, the probability of a driving event to produce a crash increases, on the average.

The distribution of driving events by BAC is limited by the maximum BAC that could occur given the amount of alcohol consumed on a drinking occasion. For example, consider the male age group 21–25. On a three-drink occasion, the average maximum possible BAC is approximately 0.09%. Even on a three-drink occasion, the BAC for a number of driving events will be at or near zero due to such factors as rate of alcohol absorption, age and body weight of the drinker, and amount of food consumed. The frequency of driving may decrease with increasing BAC due to severe impairment of the driver. Driving events at BAC=0.09% or greater will be less frequent on average, as they occur only when the drinker consumes three drinks rapidly on an empty stomach and immediately drives.

The empirical distribution of driving events as a function of BAC is different for each consumption class and, of course, varies from community to community and culture to culture. Not only do higher consumption classes have more driving events involving alcohol, but the associated average BAC is higher as well. The distribution of driving events as a function of BAC can be represented as a family of curves – one curve for each consumption class or for each age and gender subgroup within a consumption class. The following characteristics influence the shapes of the curves for each age-gender-consumption class subgroup:

- The number of driving events per capita within any age and gender group is independent of the alcohol consumption pattern. (In the aggregate, heavy drinkers, light drinkers, and non-drinkers are assumed to drive equal numbers of trips.)
- A drinking event is often followed by driving, particularly if little public transportation is available as in the US or Australia. However, the probability of a non-zero-BAC driving event is influenced by the fact that alcohol is most often consumed at night, particularly on weekend nights, whereas most driving occurs during the day on weekdays.
- Zero-BAC driving events are the most frequent driving events in every consumption class.
- The frequency of zero-BAC driving events decreases with increasing consumption class; it is highest for consumption class 1 and lowest for consumption class 4.
- Within a consumption class, the frequencies of driving events consistently decrease with increasing BAC; the distribution has no secondary peaks.
- At any given BAC resulting from a drinking occasion, heavier drinkers (consumption classes 3 and 4) may be more likely to drive than consumption classes 1 or 2.
- The incidence of drinking and driving increases between ages 13 and 33 and declines thereafter.
- Within a given age group, men are much more likely than women to drink and drive. This may be the result of gender-differentiated driving patterns; women generally drive far less than men, and so have fewer driving trips per capita. However, other factors may be involved.

An example of an approach to modeling drinking and driving events comes from the *SimCom* model, which distributes per capita driving events for each of 56 age-gender-consumption subgroups (14 age-gender groups × four consumption classes) across six BAC ranges, as shown in Fig. 6.2. The ranges for the six BAC groups are as follows: 0.0% (BAC1), >0 but <0.05% (BAC2), 0.05% to < 0.08% (BAC3), 0.08% to <0.10% (BAC4), 0.10% to <0.15% (BAC5), and ≤0.15% (BAC6).

The distribution of drinks per occasion (DPO) for a given age-gender-consumption subgroup determines the distribution of driving events as a function of the driver's BAC for that subgroup. The distribution of driving events by BAC for a given age-gender-consumption subgroup ranges from 0.0 to 0.15% BAC. From this distribution, the number of driving events in each BAC range for a particular subgroup can be estimated. In *SimCom*,

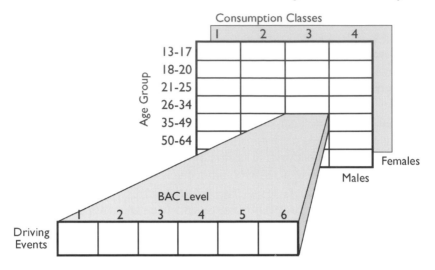

Figure 6.2 Distribution of driving events by age, sex, consumption class, and BAC level.

the distribution of driving events by BAC for a given age-gender-consumption subgroup is described by the following equation:

$$\ln y = a + bx + c \left(\sqrt{x}\right) \text{ or } y = e^{(a + bx + c(\sqrt{x}))}$$

where y is the probability of a driving event at BAC level x, e is the base of the natural system of logarithms, and a, b, and c are parameters empirically determined from data on driving patterns and alcohol consumption patterns in the US.

Such distributions are dynamic, changing to reflect changes in variables that affect BAC distributions or driving patterns for each subgroup, such as the distribution of DPO, the average number of driving trips and average distance per trip, or the perceived risk of arrest for drinking and driving. As these variables change, the three parameters are changed to describe a new distribution that reflects the influence of these variables on drinking and driving.

Legal definition of drinking and driving

When driving after or while drinking is made illegal, formal definitions of an illegal status are often established. Legal definitions of drinking and driving in a community may range from officer judgment about driver impairment to precisely measured BAC. Before reliable technology for measuring BAC was developed, the sole definition of drunk driving was officer judgment of the driver's impairment. Such a definition allows wide discretion by the officer, in selective enforcement (determining whom to stop), in the signs used to determine whether the driver has been drinking (such as slurred speech or smell of alcohol), and in the behaviors used to indicate impairment (such as body sway while walking a straight line or poor hand-to-eye coordination). In general, driver behavior has to be extreme to be defined by the officer as "drunk driving."

In many industrialized cultures, officer discretion has in recent years been reduced, and impairment has come to be defined by the BAC measured at the time the driver is stopped by the police. A legal BAC limit is set, at or above which the driver is judged legally impaired for driving and can be charged with a crime. Because the use of a BAC limit as the criterion for impairment is a legal compromise, limits often have been set at levels where drivers would appear obviously impaired. In response to recent declines in tolerance of drinking and driving, some cultures have set low BAC limits; for example, the limit in Sweden is 0.02%. However, many countries still do not set BAC limits for drinking and driving, but continue to rely on officer judgment.

Level of DUI enforcement

Enforcement of laws against drinking and driving is reflected in arrests for DUI or driving while impaired (DWI). (This discussion uses the term "DUI.") In any community, the probability that a driver who has been drinking will be stopped is very low. Thus, the number of DUI arrests in a given year is the product of the number of officers engaged in DUI enforcement and the average number of arrests per officer. A number of factors may affect the per-officer arrest rate in a given community.

The most obvious factor affecting the per-officer arrest rate is the priority law enforcement officials place on DUI enforcement. In most US states, arrests per officer have increased since the early 1970s, as DUI enforcement has been given a higher priority. DUI arrests take considerable officer time, as officers must detect impaired drivers, collect evidence, and testify in court. Breathalyzers (equipment for measuring BAC by sampling exhaled breath) have decreased the time it takes to make a DUI arrest. As breathalyzers have improved and become more available, officers have become more inclined to make DUI arrests and more efficient in making them.

An enforcement strategy that can increase the DUI arrest rate is the use of special DUI patrols. With no other enforcement tasks to perform, DUI patrols can make many more arrests in a given period of time than routine patrols can. For instance, Jonah & Wilson (1983) reported that in Australia, random police checkpoints reduced the number of drivers on the road with high BACs. However, without measures of the total number of driving events, it cannot be known whether this change represents redistribution of drivers to lower BACs or reduction of the number of drivers on the road. Whitehead (1975) argued that lowering the BAC limit will redistribute the entire spectrum of drivers to lower BAC levels. However, Jonah & Wilson (1983) contended that any deterrent effects are likely to occur only among moderate drinkers.

A study of drivers in Finland following the imposition of random breath testing found a decrease in the number of drivers with positive BACs at both low and high levels (Dunbar, Penttila & Pikkarainen, 1987). These investigators noted that the incidence of high BACs was highest between 7:00 A.M. and 10:00 A.M., because drivers are generally unaware how long it takes to eliminate alcohol from the body. Therefore, a reduction in total DUI would seem more likely to result from overall moderation of drinking and driving behavior than from simply forcing intoxicated persons to avoid driving. (For a further discussion of the effects of special enforcement, see Homel, 1988, 1993, in Australia; and Voas & Hause, 1987, in the US.)

In summary, a community's level of DUI enforcement is reflected in the number of DUI arrests made per officer, which depends on the capability of local law enforcement to detect and arrest DUI offenders, and the priority given to DUI enforcement by local law enforcement authorities and/or the community.

Actual vs. perceived risk of arrest and sanction for drinking and driving

Deterrence of drinking and driving through DUI enforcement depends primarily on drivers' perceptions of their risk of arrest for DUI, which in turn depend not only on the actual risk of arrest, but on the legal BAC limit (which affects both perceived and actual risk), the level of public attention to DUI enforcement, and changes in any of these factors.

In most communities, the actual risk of arrest for drinking and driving is quite low. In the US, it has been estimated that approximately one arrest is made for every 2000 driving events above the legal BAC limit (Borkenstein, 1975). Ross (1982) analyzed the effects of the British Road Safety Act of 1967, which provided for mandatory BAC tests and defined driving with a BAC of 0.08% as a *per se* offense. Implementation of the act was accompanied by a massive publicity campaign. Ross found that the act did not greatly increase the actual risk of DUI arrest in the event of drinking and driving; rather, it changed drivers' perceptions of the risk of arrest. Ross concluded that perceived risk can be a most powerful factor in deterrence of drinking and driving.

People learn from experience when the chance of getting caught is small. When perceived risk of arrest for DUI is high, people are less likely, on average, to drive after drinking. When perceived risk of arrest is low, DUI enforcement has little or no deterrent effect, and drinking and driving behavior seeks a natural limit, based on actual risk of arrest. Modest changes in the actual risk of arrest are unlikely to have much effect on driver behavior (Reed,1981; Ross, 1982). However, substantially bolstering DUI enforcement, though effective (Voas & Hause, 1987), can be politically and economically costly.

Increasing perceived risk is an important means of reducing drinking and driving. Risk compensation theory (Peltzman, 1975; Wilde, 1982) suggests that if people perceive risk of arrest for DUI as increasing, they will seek to reduce their own risk to an acceptable threshold by, for example, driving more carefully after drinking or drinking less before driving. However, large changes in perceived risk are needed to significantly reduce drinking and driving behavior.

In the short run, when changes in enforcement are implemented, and especially when they are well publicized, the public generally overestimates the increased risk – at least for a time, as in the British public's reduction in drinking and driving following implementation of the British Road Safety Act of 1967. However, when it became clear that the actual risk of arrest had not actually risen appreciably, the English driving public adjusted its behavior accordingly, and drinking and driving increased again, tending toward their former levels (Ross, 1982).

Similarly, in a study of a three-year program of special DUI patrols in Stockton, California, Voas & Hause (1987) found that the risk of arrest for DUI increased nearly ten-fold and that alcohol-involved crashes declined after news coverage brought public attention to this increased risk of arrest. As publicity declined, the actual risk of arrest remained at this higher level, but alcohol-involved crashes began to increase. By the time the special three-year patrol program was over, alcohol-involved crash rates had returned to their prior levels. Drinking and driving behavior had been affected more by drivers' perceptions of their risk of arrest, resulting from news coverage, than by the actual risk.

If DUI enforcement increases substantially enough, perceived risk may increase even without an increase in news coverage or other publicity. For example, when random breath testing was introduced into New South Wales, Australia, the actual risk of detection greatly increased, resulting in increased perceived risk, and alcohol-involved arrests and crashes declined (Homel, 1993). There was no sustained publicity of random breath testing, but the deterrence effect held due to highly visible enforcement.

Ross (1983) suggested that many individuals at high risk for drinking and driving (e.g., problem drinkers and youths) may not accurately evaluate their levels of impairment. In fact, drivers in general poorly estimate their BAC or degree of impairment (Beirness, 1984; Clayton, 1986; Russ, Harwood & Geller, 1986). Thus, in the absence of factors that would increase perceived risk, this tendency to underestimate impairment may cause drivers (especially those at high risk for drinking and driving) to underestimate their actual risk of arrest for DUI.

Drinking and driving behavior is also affected by the perceived risk of punishment (sanctions) following arrest. Sanctions are established by the community for two purposes: to penalize violations of the law; and to deter future violations by the offender or others through the threat of punishment. Sanctions for those convicted of DUI have included fines, jail, and loss of driver's license. The greater the certainty of conviction and the more severe the punishment, the more effective sanctions are in deterring drinking and driving behavior. Severe sanctions provide little or no deterrence if the likelihood of conviction is small. Ross (1985) has noted that the deterrent effect results from the certainty of punishment, rather than its severity. In fact, he documented that in states and localities that enact stricter penalties for DUI, the conviction rates tend to drop. There is evidence (reviewed by Edwards et al., 1994) that the threat of mandatory license suspension has a general deterrent effect.

The effect of public attention to DUI enforcement on perceived risk

When changes in traffic enforcement are well publicized, the public tends to overestimate the new, increased risk – at least for a time – and drinking and driving declines. When it becomes clear that the actual risk of arrest has not risen appreciably, the public perception of risk reverts to its former level (reflecting actual risk), and drinking and driving increases. Figure 6.3 illustrates the influence of publicity on the relationship between actual and perceived risk of DUI arrest. In the absence of publicity about DUI enforcement, perceived risk seeks the level of actual risk, about which it oscillates. Publicity about enforcement efforts may temporarily cause per-

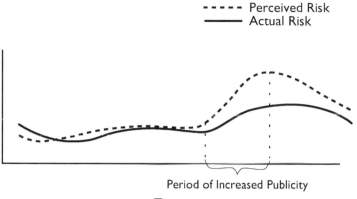

Figure 6.3 Perceived risk of arrest increasing dramatically in a period of high publicity.

ceived risk to exceed actual risk. However, after a rapid rise, perceived risk will gradually decay to approximate actual risk.

Public attention to DUI enforcement depends on the coverage or publicity given to this issue in the news media or other public information sources. To sustain a given level of perceived risk of DUI arrest (above the actual risk level), some maintenance level of annual news coverage of the issue is required.

An indicator of the level of news coverage, such as the annual number of newspaper articles about drinking and driving, can be used as a relative indicator of community attention to DUI enforcement. For example, 200 news articles per year in one daily newspaper would indicate a higher level of attention than 50 articles. Of course, article counts are crude indicators of actual public attention, because they do not account for article length, accompanying headlines and photographs, or page placement. However, the latter characteristics of coverage are less easily quantified than article counts.

The effects of a change in public attention to DUI enforcement depend on both the absolute level of attention and the size of the change. For example, if 200 articles per year indicates a "high" level of community attention to DUI enforcement, then the level after a 10% decrease (to 180 articles) is still relatively high. If 50 articles per year indicates "moderate" or even "low" attention, then a 10% decrease (to 45 articles) may represent a significant decrease in public attention. Table 6.1 illustrates the potential relative strength of effect on public attention associated with changes in

Table 6.1. *Illustration of relative effects of changes*
in news coverage on public attention

Local DUI news coverage (articles/year)	Annual change (%)	Strength of effect on public attention
50	+1	Moderate increase
	−1	Moderate increase
100	−1	Unchanged (remains moderate)
200	−1	Unchanged (remains moderate)

news coverage of DUI enforcement. In this example, a 1% increase (or decrease) from a level of 50 articles per year has a greater effect on public attention than a 1% percent increase (or decrease) from 200 articles per year.

Figure 6.4 illustrates a possible relationship between public attention to DUI enforcement (measured as news coverage) and perceived risk of DUI arrest. In period A, news coverage is assumed to be zero, and perceived risk is fairly close to actual risk. In period B, actual enforcement remains stable, but news coverage of (and thus public attention to) DUI enforcement substantially increases, causing a large increase in perceived risk. As long as news coverage is greater than zero, perceived risk remains higher than actual risk. Without additional news coverage, perceived risk declines over time. In period C, news coverage of DUI enforcement decreases, and perceived risk decreases to a level lower than in period B but higher than in period A. (Note that in this example, actual risk does not change.)

Influence of the legal BAC limit on perceived risk

Setting of a BAC limit not only provides a basis for legal sanctions, but also serves as a deterrent. As the BAC limit is lowered, drivers are deterred, on average, from driving after drinking, because the likelihood of their exceeding the lower BAC level is higher, and thus their actual risk of arrest and conviction for DUI is increased. When a decrease in the BAC limit results in an increase in the arrest rate for DUI, perceived risk will increase sharply, and then (in the absence of other stimuli) decay to match the new

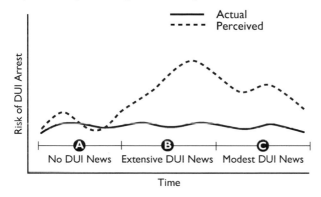

Figure 6.4 Illustration of relationship of DUI news coverage and actual DUI enforcement to perceived risk of DUI detection and arrest.

level of enforcement (i.e., the new actual risk of arrest). The amount by which perceived risk abruptly increases depends on the magnitude of the change in the BAC limit and the level at which the new limit is set. In other words, the greater the decrease in the BAC limit and/or the lower the new BAC limit, the greater the increase in perceived risk.

When the BAC limit is lowered, the change in perceived risk of arrest can be conceived as an increment over the previously stable level, as illustrated in Fig. 6.5. The first part of the time-series curve (labeled "A") shows perceived risk oscillating around a stable actual risk of arrest when the legal driving limit for BAC is 0.10%. The second part of the series (labeled "B") shows that when the legal limit is lowered to 0.08%, perceived risk increases sharply, as does the actual DUI arrest risk. In the third part of the time-series (labeled "C"), perceived risk declines to a level higher than the former stable level and closer to the new actual risk of arrest.

The dynamics of drinking and driving

The three empirically determined parameters (a, b, and c) of the functional form for drinking and driving have been defined in *SimCom*. They depend on the community's driving and drinking patterns, and the effects on these patterns of the perceived risk of arrest and conviction for DUI. Drivers' perceived risk of sanctions for DUI is a major variable influencing drinking and driving behavior. Perceived risk may change as a result of changes in public attention to DUI enforcement, the level of DUI enforcement, the legal BAC limit, or the severity of sanctions for DUI. The actual risk of arrest is a function of DUI enforcement capacity and the BAC limit.

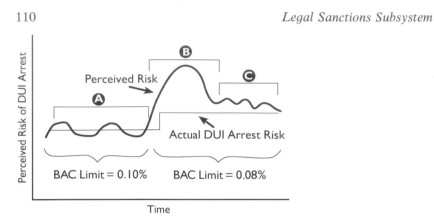

Figure 6.5 Illustration of relationship of BAC legal limit and perceived risk of DUI detection and arrest.

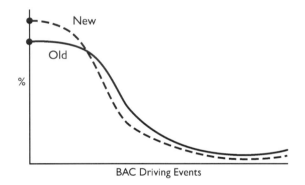

Figure 6.6 Example of shift in drink/drive distribution in response to perceived risk increase.

When perceived risk of DUI arrest or drinks per occasion change in ways that lower the frequency of drinking and driving, zero-BAC driving events become more frequent (i.e., the y-intercept of the curve is raised). The numbers of non-zero-BAC driving events also decrease, changing the shape of the curve. Figure 6.6 illustrates this effect of an increase in perceived risk on the distribution of driving events as a function of BAC.

Interaction with other subsystems

The dynamics of the Legal Sanctions Subsystem and its interactions with other subsystems are illustrated in Fig. 6.7. The Legal Sanctions Subsystem

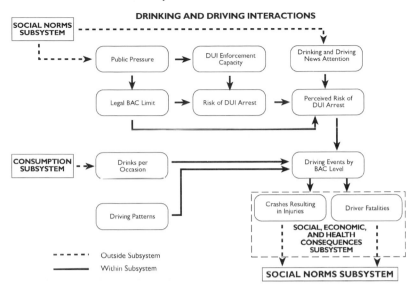

Figure 6.7 Drinking and driving within the Legal Sanctions Subsystem.

reflects the use of local police powers to enforce specific laws concerning
alcohol purchase, and drinking locations and activities (including total
bans on sale of alcohol). In some cases, the enforcement roles of the Formal
Regulation and Control Subsystem and the Legal Sanctions Subsystem
overlap. Although the Formal Regulation and Control Subsystem establishes the laws and rules concerning retail sale of alcohol and drinking in
other locations or situations (e.g., public intoxication or drinking and
driving), enforcement of these laws locally can also be the domain of the
Legal Sanctions Subsystem. Enforcement activities within the Formal
Regulation and Control Subsystem most often are limited to licensing of
retail alcohol outlets and monitoring their compliance with rules governing their operations (such as rules against sales to underage persons or to
obviously intoxicated patrons). In many US communities, local police
share responsibility with state alcoholic beverage control (ABC) officers for
enforcement of laws regulating sale of alcohol.

The Legal Sanctions Subsystem is influenced by the Social Norms
Subsystem through community concern about specific alcohol-involved
problems, and public pressure for enforcement of laws related to alcohol
sales and drinking behavior. For example, the level of DUI enforcement
(i.e., the number of officers made available for DUI enforcement efforts,
and the rates of prosecution and/or conviction for drinking and driving)

reflects public pressure for enforcement through the Social Norms Subsystem. Intoxication within one's residence may be socially acceptable, but intoxication in public places may be unacceptable; if the level of community concern about public intoxication is high, laws against this behavior may be vigorously enforced.

Changes in the community's drinking patterns, manifested in the Consumption Subsystem, may result in changes in the probability (likelihood) that individuals will drink in a prohibited manner, e.g., drive with a given BAC. Of considerable influence are general drinking patterns (discussed in Chapter 2), which can be affected by factors such as income, demographic characteristics of the community, the price of alcoholic beverages, local alcohol availability and promotion, and cultural changes that reflect changes in values and drinking norms.

The problem of drinking and driving provides a significant example of how the Legal Sanctions Subsystem interacts with other subsystems. Within a community, the distribution of driving events by the driver's BAC is influenced by community alcohol consumption level and drinking patterns. These in turn are influenced by social norms for acceptable levels of drinking (especially in conjunction with driving). The Social Norms Subsystem also influences the intensity and severity of enforcement of laws against drinking and driving. In turn, alcohol use in conjunction with driving affects the Social, Economic, and Health Consequences Subsystem, particularly through alcohol-involved automobile crashes. Similar dynamics exist for other alcohol-involved behaviors, such as public drunkenness or violence.

7

Social, Economic, and Health Consequences Subsystem: community identification of and responses to alcohol problems

Introduction

The use of alcohol can have a wide range of social, economic, and health consequences in a community. Some of these consequences, such as liver cirrhosis or alcohol psychosis and resulting hospitalizations, may result from long-term use of alcohol. Other consequences may result from the heavy use of alcohol on occasions where impairment in judgment, function, or physical skills results in injury or death of the drinker or others, and emergency medical services may be required.

Alcohol increases the risks of all types of injury or violence. For example, the frequency with which drinking and violence towards a spouse co-occur indicates that alcohol increases the risk of spouse abuse. Not all cases of spouse abuse are caused by drinking; however, the acute effects of alcohol may increase violent or victim behavior of either spouse, or violence towards a spouse may be precipitated by family disruption associated with long-term or heavy dependent drinking. Examples of accidents made more likely by alcohol impairment include motor vehicle crashes and drownings.

The Social, Economic, and Health Consequences Subsystem has three functions in the community:

(1) Definition and identification of alcohol-involved problems.
(2) Remedial or preventive response to these problems.
(3) Direction of public attention to these problems.

It is not always obvious what constitutes an alcohol-involved problem for the community. The seemingly trivial case of a hangover from drinking illustrates the subtlety of some alcohol-involved problems. Most experienced drinkers have had hangovers, and hangovers have been the subject of many comedy routines; this drinking-related outcome is not generally considered a community problem. However, if an employee cannot come to work or causes an accident at work as a result of a hangover, then a hangover could be defined as an alcohol-involved problem. Family violence provides an example of a more serious unrecognized problem. For many years, family violence was not publicly discussed, and many spouses (especially women) were unable to leave abusive situations, either for fear or for economic reasons. In recent years, in industrialized countries, the issue of family violence has become more public and has come to be defined as a problem, and the role of alcohol in family violence is more recognized in the community.

Community identification of an alcohol-involved problem is not necessarily based on the frequency of the event. For example, birth defects resulting from the mother's drinking during pregnancy, such as fetal alcohol syndrome (FAS), are relatively rare; one recent estimate of their frequency is 0.33 FAS cases per 1000 live births (Abel & Sokol, 1991). However, the high level of social concern about infants has resulted in considerable public attention to the problem. See discussion of salience in Chapter 5. The US has established a nationally mandated warning label concerning the risk of drinking during pregnancy, and some communities have established similar locally mandated warning labels (enforced by the Formal Regulation and Control Subsystem).

In some cases, definition and identification may be the community's only response to an alcohol-involved problem. For example, although alcohol often is present in the blood of homicide victims, the role of alcohol in victimization has rarely been addressed by a preventive or remedial community response; murder is viewed as a criminal justice problem, not an alcohol-involved problem.

The community's remedial action in response to alcohol-involved problems and behaviors (other than law-enforcement responses through the Legal Sanctions Subsystem) includes provision of social and health services via the Social, Economic, and Health Consequences Subsystem. The demand for community social and health services can be strongly related to alcohol use. For example, a person who has been drinking and is injured in a fall will be treated in the local emergency room or trauma center, as part of the community's health-services response. Many hospital admissions and emergency-room visits are directly or indirectly related to alcohol use. Social and health services also include detoxification and recovery treatment for alcohol dependency or alcoholism.

The Social, Economic, and Health Consequences Subsystem also makes public alcohol-involved events (such as deaths or injuries caused by drinking and driving), which in turn can increase community concern about such problems, through the Social Norms Subsystem. For example, if injuries caused by alcohol-involved violence are increasing in the community, community concern about this problem is nonetheless unlikely to increase unless the problem is publicly recognized (e.g., in newspaper coverage, published statistics, announcements by officials, or attention from special-interest groups). If public attention is brought to this trend, community concern can increase, resulting in community demands for response to the problem. See discussion of news media attention to alcohol-involved events in Chapter 5.

This chapter first discusses issues in identification of alcohol-involved problems, including the concepts of individual and aggregate risk, and the classification of types of alcohol-involved problems. It then categorizes community responses to alcohol-involved problems, and the economic consequences of the problems and the responses. Finally, interactions of the Social, Economic, and Health Consequences Subsystem with other subsystems are summarized.

Identification of alcohol-involved events as problems

In general, an event or process becomes defined as a "problem" if the community considers it to be undesirable. Alcohol-involved problems in the Social, Economic, and Health Consequences Subsystem are events or situations judged to disrupt the natural functioning of a specific sector or subsystem of the community, and whose frequency or risk of occurrence is increased by use of alcohol. These problems typically involve disruption of the workplace or family, threats to personal health and safety, or threats to public values and decorum. They can also include intentional violence, such as assault, murder, suicide, or intentional self-injury (such as poisoning or mutilation).

Short-term consumption of alcohol can impair an individual sufficiently to increase the chance of injury or death through such events as motor vehicle crashes, drownings, burns, and falls. Injuries and fatalities from traffic and non-traffic accidents and deaths related to the use of alcohol in the event are classified as "acute morbidity and mortality." Long-term consumption of alcohol can cause potentially fatal physiological damage to the body. For example, the liver is particularly affected by ethanol (the active ingredient in alcoholic beverages), and long-term alcohol consumption can result in death from liver failure. Alcohol-related chronic diseases and deaths from such disease are classified as "chronic morbidity and

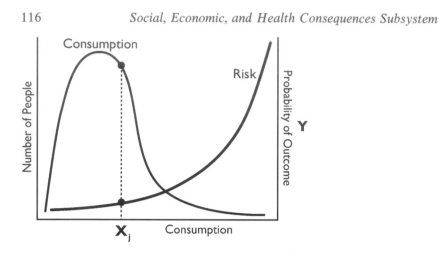

Figure 7.1 Distributions of consumption and outcome risk.

mortality." By documenting the annual alcohol-related acute and chronic morbidity and mortality, the Social, Economic, and Health Consequences Subsystem formally defines what events can be considered alcohol-involved problems. See discussion of risk distributions and alcohol consumption by Anderson (1995) and Edwards et al. (1994).

Risk of alcohol-involved problems

The risk of an alcohol-involved problem is the probability of the event occurring in association with a specific rate and pattern of alcohol consumption. In Fig. 7.1, the horizontal (X) axis is the possible range of alcohol consumption levels over a defined period (e.g., annually). The curve on the left side of the graph is a distribution of alcohol consumption; the left vertical axis is the number of people, and the height of the curve at any point (X_j) on the horizontal axis is the number of people who drink X_j amount of alcohol over a defined period (e.g., annually). The curve reaching its peak at the right edge of the graph is the distribution of risk for an outcome Y. The right vertical axis is the probability of outcome Y, and the height of the curve at any point (X_j) on the horizontal axis is the risk of that outcome among people who drink X_j amount of alcohol over the defined period.

The individual risk for outcome Y is the product of the probability of consuming a given amount of alcohol per unit time (X_j) and the probability of outcome Y at that consumption level:

Prob (outcome Y) = Prob(X_j) × Prob(Y,X_j)

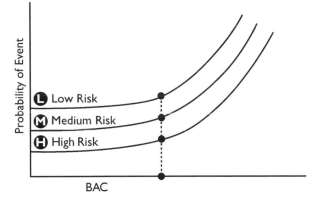

Figure 7.2 Distribution of event outcome risk by BAC.

The aggregate risk of outcome Y for a given population of individuals is expressed by this equation:

SUM (outcome Y) = SUM{NX$_j$ × ⌊Prob(X$_j$) × Prob(Y,X$_j$)]}

where N = the size of the population. In this example, aggregate risk is defined according to the amount of alcohol consumed over some specified period (such as one year or ten years). Although this formulation can be used to define the risk of any type of alcohol-involved event, it is particularly useful for defining risks of events resulting from long-term exposure to alcohol (e.g., chronic mortality, as from cirrhosis).

For events that occur not from accumulated exposure to alcohol over time, but at a particular moment (acute morbidity and mortality), the risk depends on the individual's degree of impairment on the given drinking occasion. Because impairment depends greatly on blood alcohol concentration (BAC) (as discussed in Chapter 6), the probability of the event can be plotted as a function of BAC. Figure 7.2 shows a family of curves relating risk of an event to BAC. The middle curve (M) represents the overall average risk. For most acute outcomes, the risk of the event increases disproportionately as BAC increases (i.e., the relationship of risk to BAC is not linear).

Individual risk of a given outcome at a given BAC depends on such factors as personal weight, prior drinking experience, and expectations concerning the effect of alcohol. To the extent that subgroups of the population differ in these factors, different risk distributions can be defined for different subgroups, as illustrated by the two other curves in Fig. 7.2. The top curve (L) represents the risk distribution for people with lower-than-average tolerance for alcohol and thus a higher-than-average risk at a given BAC. For example, curve L might represent the risk among young, less-experienced drinkers or among people of lower body weight. The bottom curve (H) represents the risk distribution for people with higher-than-average tolerance for alcohol and thus a lower-than-average risk at a given BAC. For example, curve H might characterize the risk among heavy drinkers or people of heavier body weight.

It is important to distinguish between individual and aggregate risk. Even if the risk of a particular outcome is positively associated with alcohol consumption for the population as a whole, the risk of that outcome can be low or zero for a given individual who has been drinking (e.g., as a result of that person's drinking experience). Conversely, even if a particular outcome is not related to alcohol consumption in the aggregate, a given individual's risk of that outcome may be increased by alcohol consumption. For example, even if there is no observed relationship between per capita alcohol consumption and occurrence of depression for the population as a whole, a particular individual may be at increasing risk for an event of depression as his or her BAC rises. The association between BAC and the risk of an outcome can differ not only among individuals but also among cultures and settings.

In addition, drinkers may not accurately perceive their own risk of incurring a drinking-related outcome. Drinkers typically underestimate their risks of drinking-related outcomes and of personal risk associated with drinking in general. Although drinkers may recognize the risk of an event at high BACs, they tend not to recognize risk at lower BACs. This tendency is illustrated in Fig. 7.3, which shows an empirically based risk curve along with an example of a potential "perceived risk" curve. The actual risk increases substantially as BAC increases. While there is risk at lower BAC levels, the drinker may not recognize this risk. In this illustration, drinkers may not perceive any risk until reaching a fairly high BAC, e.g., BAC > 1.0. Then even when drinkers begin to perceive risk, this perceived risk is substantially below the actual risk.

Perceived risk of harm or increased threat can influence behavior. In general, if one perceives that personal risk increases as more and more alcohol is consumed or in conjunction with a specific situation, then drinking can be affected. As described in the Legal Sanctions Subsystem, perceived risk of drinking and driving enforcement influences decisions about driving after drinking.

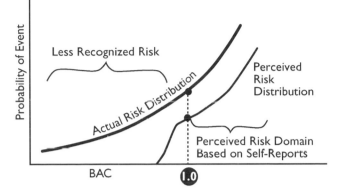

Figure 7.3 Illustration of actual risk versus perceived risk.

Alcohol-involved chronic morbidity and mortality

Alcohol-involved deaths and illnesses resulting from long-term exposure to alcohol are most likely to affect long-term heavy drinkers. Within the Social, Economic, and Health Consequences Subsystem, chronic disease morbidity and mortality are coded according to the International Classification of Disease (ICD), which was developed by the World Health Organization, and typically is used in hospital admissions and on death certificates. Table 7.1 shows the alcohol-related causes of death in the ICD Version 8 (used through 1978) and Version 9 (used since 1979).

Heavy alcohol use increases the overall risk of mortality. The association between increased alcohol consumption and increased risk of mortality from certain alcohol-related chronic diseases is well documented. Cirrhosis of the liver, the most common of these, increases sharply with regular consumption. Norström (1987) found a strong association using time-series data in Sweden between per capita consumption and cirrhosis mortality. A similar result was obtained in an analysis of Danish mortality (Thorsen, 1990). In a ten-year study of 8060 health-care patients in the US, Klatsky, Friedman & Siegelaub (1981) found that those who averaged three to five drinks per day ran a risk of cirrhosis nearly twice that of abstainers and occasional drinkers. Those who averaged six or more drinks per day were six times as likely to be diagnosed with the disease as abstainers and occasional drinkers. Among the respondents in a follow-up survey of more than 275 000 US men aged 40 to 59, Boffetta & Garfinkel (1990) found an even greater increase in risk. Occasional drinkers are 50% more likely to die of cirrhosis than non-drinkers. The likelihood of death from cirrhosis

Table 7.1. *Alcohol-related codes from the ICD*

VERSION 8	VERSION 9
Alcoholic psychoses 291	*Alcoholic psychoses 291*
291.0 Delirium Tremens	291.0 Alcohol Withdrawal Delirium
291.1 Korsakov's Psychosis	291.1 Alcohol Amnestic Syndrome
291.2 Other Alcoholic Hallucinosis	291.2 Other Alcoholic Dementia
291.3 Alcoholic Paranoid	291.3 Alcohol Withdrawal Hallucinosis
291.4 to 291.8 Not present	291.4 Idiosyncratic Alcohol Intoxication
291.9 Other and Unspecified	291.5 Alcoholic Jealousy
Alcoholic:	*291.6–291.7 Not present*
dementia	291.8 Other Specific Alcoholic Psychosis
insanity	291.9 Unspecified Alcoholic Psychosis
NOS or of any type not classifiable	
under 291.0–291.3	*Alcohol dependency syndrome 303*
mania	303.0 Acute Alcoholic Intoxication
psychosis	*303.1 to 303.8 Not present*
	303.9 Other and Unspecified Alcohol
Alcoholism 303	Dependence
303.0 Episodic Excessive Drinking	
303.1 Habitual Excessive Drinking	*Non-dependent abuse of drugs 305*
303.2 Alcoholic Addiction	305.0 Alcohol Abuse
303.3 to 303.8 Not present	305.00 Unspecified
303.9 Other and Unspecified Alcoholism	305.01 Continuous
	305.02 Episodic
	305.03 In Remission
	Inflammatory and toxic neuropathy 357
	357.5 Alcoholic Polyneuropathy
	Cardiomyopathy 425
	425.5 Alcoholic Cardiomyopathy
	Gastritis and duodenitis 535
	535.3 Alcoholic Gastritis
Cirrhosis with or without mention of alcohol 571	*Cirrhosis with or without mention of alcohol 571*
571.0 Alcoholic	*listed as Chronic Liver diseases and cirrhosis 571*
	571.0 Alcoholic Fatty Liver
571.1 to 571.8 Not present	571.1 Acute Alcoholic Hepatitis
	571.2 Alcoholic Cirrhosis of Liver
571.9 Other – without mention of alcohol or	571.3 Alcoholic Liver Damage, Unspecified
alcoholism	571.4 Chronic Hepatitis
	571.40 Chronic hepatitis, unspecified
	571.41 Chronic persistent hepatitis
	571.49 Other:
	Chronic hepatitis
	active
	aggressive
	Recurrent hepatitis
	571.5 Cirrhosis of Liver without mention of
	Alcohol
	571.6 Biliary Cirrhosis
	571.7 Not present
	571.8 Other Chronic Non-alcoholic Liver
	Diseases
	571.9 Unspecified Chronic Liver Disease
	without mention of Alcohol
	Liver abscess and sequelae of chronic liver
	diseases 572
	572.3 Portal Hypertension
	Non-specific findings on examination of blood 790
	790.3 Excessive Blood Level of Alcohol
Toxic effect of ethyl alcohol	*Toxic effect of alcohol 980*
N980.0 Ethyl Alcohol not N980.1 or .2 or .9	980.0 Ethyl Alcohol
Accidental alcohol poisoning	*Accidental poisoning by alcohol, not elsewhere*
E860 Accidental Poisoning by Alcohol	*classified E860*
(No decimal codes)	E860.0 Alcoholic Beverages
	E860.1 Other and Unspecified Ethyl
	Alcohol and its Products

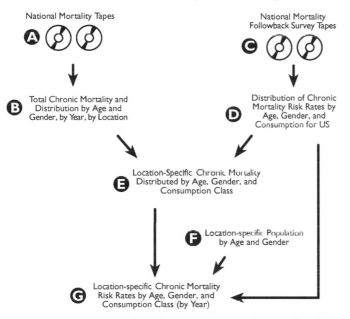

Figure 7.4 Derivation of location-specific chronic mortality risk rates by age, gender, and consumption class.

among men who average three drinks per day is five times that of abstainers and three times that of occasional drinkers. Among men who average six or more drinks per day, the likelihood of death from cirrhosis is 12 times that of occasional drinkers and 18 times that of non-drinkers.

Figure 7.4 illustrates how risk distributions (such as those used in *SimCom*) for chronic mortality by age, gender, and consumption class can be derived from data available for the US. The National Mortality Data (A) gives chronic mortality by age and gender, by year (B). The National Mortality Followback Survey (NMFS) (C) provides a distribution of chronic mortality by age, gender, and consumption class. The NMFS was an effort to develop estimates of the quantity or frequency of alcohol consumption for each dead person. From these data, a risk matrix (D) can be developed that provides estimated relative risk for chronic mortality by age and gender group for each of four consumption classes. This distribution can be applied to (B) for a specific location, to redistribute total chronic mortality by age, gender, and consumption class (E). Dividing the location-specific population by age and gender (F) into (E) provides a location-specific distribution of chronic mortality risk rates by age, gender, and consumption class (G). Theoretically, the same process could be used to develop a similar distribution of chronic morbidity risk; however, informa-

tion on alcohol consumption by age and gender is not routinely collected
for hospitalized patients in the US or most other countries.

Alcohol-involved acute morbidity and mortality

The risk of injury or death resulting from sudden or unexpected events can
be increased by short-term consumption of alcohol. Alcohol can impair
motor skills, cognition, and the ability to respond to difficult or emergency
situations. The most important causes of alcohol-involved acute morbidity
and mortality are accidents (motor-vehicle-related or not). Alcohol also
can increase the risk of injuries or death resulting from intentional action.
Certain events and types of injuries are particularly related to BAC. For
example, alcohol is detected in the blood more often and at higher levels
among victims of road accidents or assaults and people with head injuries
than among other injury victims (Wechsler et al., 1969; Holt et al., 1980;
Joksch, 1985).

Traffic fatalities and injuries are deaths of drivers, passengers, or pedestrians resulting from motor vehicle crashes. For example, in the US, 40 to
50% of traffic fatalities result from accidents involving drivers who have
been drinking (Zador et al., 1988; Zobeck, et al., 1991). *Non-traffic accidental fatalities and injuries* are deaths and injuries resulting from events that
do not involve motor vehicles; these include burns, falls, drownings or
near-drownings, boating accidents, poisonings, choking, lacerations, and
accidental discharge of firearms. Alcohol use increases the risk of many of
these causes of death (Hingson & Howland, 1987; Howland & Hingson,
1987; Saltz, Gruenewald & Hennessy, 1992).

Studies of emergency-room populations have shown that injured patients are likely to have detectable blood alcohol levels. Cherpitel &
Rosovsky (1990) found such a relationship in Mexico, Cherpitel (1988,
1992, 1994) in the US, and Honkanen et al. (1983) in Finland found that the
risk of injury increases with increasing BAC. See Cherpitel (1993) for a
review of international studies of alcohol and injury. In a literature review,
Howland & Hingson (1987) found that victims of fires and burns are likely
to have alcohol in their blood; however, actual risk rates vary widely across
studies. A similar relationship exists for drownings (Howland & Hingson,
1988). Drinking patterns are related to the risk of mortality. For example,
Anda, Williamson & Remington (1988) found that persons who on average
consume five or more drinks per occasion are nearly twice as likely to die of
fatal injuries than persons who drink less.

The role of alcohol in non-intentional home, recreational, and occupational injuries has been demonstrated by Smith & Kraus (1988) and Honkanen (1993), who found that one to two-thirds of people injured in non-traffic accidents have detectable BACs. Studies indicate that alcohol use is an important factor in home and recreational injuries. In contrast, associations between in-the-event alcohol exposure and occupational injuries have been inconsistent (Lagerlof, Valverius & Westerholm, 1984; Hingson, Lederman & Walsh, 1985), possibly because information on exposure associated with occupational injury is lacking (Smith & Kraus, 1988).

Intentional injuries and deaths (i.e., resulting from intentional actions) are considered to be alcohol-involved if either the perpetrator or the victim had been drinking and the drinking increased the risk of the violent act. Such events include both child or spouse abuse (i.e., physical injury or sexual assault on a child or a spouse by a family member) and non-family violence, such as fights, assaults, and attacks away from home. In general, the role of alcohol in assaults is to increase the role of violence, all other things being equal (Parker, 1995).

Two types of acute deaths are considered intentional: homicide and suicide. Studies in the US have shown that approximately 50% of homicide victims have been drinking at the time of death (Wolfgang, 1958; Parker & Rebhun, 1995) and that a larger percentage of people who commit crimes have been drinking (Collins, 1981). Suicide also has a significant level of alcohol involvement, but it is not known whether drinking is a causal factor in death or whether victims consume alcohol to prepare for death. A link between alcohol and suicide has been found in France (Norström, 1988), Hungary (Skog & Elekes, 1993), and Norway and Sweden (Rossow, 1993).

Other alcohol-involved problems

Other alcohol-involved problems occur in the workplace, the home (in addition to child or spouse abuse), and public locations.

Workplace problems are events relating to the ability to successfully perform tasks on the job, injury of oneself or others at the workplace, or destruction of workplace property (as discussed by Roman, 1990). The following events are examples of alcohol-involved workplace problems:

- Self-reported work disruptions: drinkers' own reports of drinking-related problems with employees, discipline, performance, or other aspects of work.

- Absences: drinking-related absences from work.
- Lowered work performance: reduction in the ability to perform assigned tasks or duties as a result of drinking.
- Workers' compensation: earnings lost as a result of work-related problems involving drinking.
- Disability compensation: disability payments to workers whose disabilities are related to drinking.
- Work accidents: injuries, death, and property damage caused by employees who have been drinking.

Family disruptions are stress, disturbances, or discord related to drinking by one or more family members and not resulting in injuries or death. Included in this category are disturbances in the family related to a family member's drinking as reported to social workers, physicians, or health professionals. Another example is divorce for reasons related to drinking by one or both spouses.

Public disruptions are public disturbances or unacceptable public behavior related to drinking in public, or drinking at or near public establishments. Examples are public intoxication and drinking-related noise, litter, gang behavior, and rowdiness.

Relationship of consumption level, drinks per occasion, impairment, and acute outcomes

Accidental injury and death as outputs from the community system can be estimated from the risk of an outcome as a function of BAC (a surrogate for impairment). For each consumption class, the expected distribution of drinks per occasion (DPO) can be used to estimate the expected distribution of BAC for each drinking occasion (as discussed in Chapter 2). The expected BAC distribution is used to calculate the expected number of alcohol-involved acute outcomes per drinking event. ·

Prevention interventions can potentially reduce both the overall level of consumption and the expected DPO for any or all consumption classes. Figure 7.5 illustrates an approach to modeling the effects of changes in consumption level or DPO distribution on the annual numbers of acute trauma events (injuries or deaths). Each DPO distribution (I) is associated with an expected BAC distribution (II). Each drinking event at a given BAC has an associated risk of an acute trauma event; the distribution of this risk by age and gender is shown as III. The product of the BAC distribution for an age and gender group (II) and the trauma risk distribu-

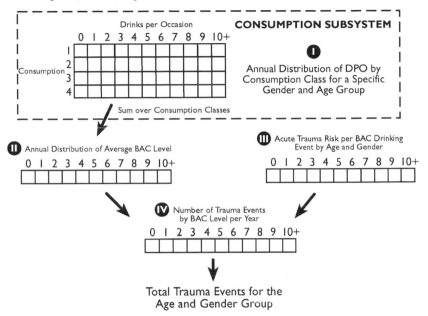

Figure 7.5 Flow chart: trauma event calculation by gender and age group between the Consumption and the Social, Economic, and Health Consequences Subsystems.

tion for that group (III) is the estimated annual number of acute trauma events for each BAC range for that age and gender group (IV). The estimates for each BAC range can be summed to estimate the total annual number of acute trauma events for that age and gender group

Where BAC is regularly measured following acute mortality, death certificate information can be used to empirically estimate acute mortality risks as a function of BAC, in an approach similar to that shown in Fig. 7.4 for chronic mortality. However, BAC data usually are not regularly collected for non-fatal injuries. Non-fatal injuries span a considerable range of severity and may be treated at a wide range of facility types (or not treated at all). The usefulness of medical facilities as sources of data on BAC related to injuries is affected by patients' decisions on whether or where to seek treatment and the facilities' BAC testing practices (see Telpin, Abram & Michaels, 1989; Cherpitel, 1993).

The least severe (and probably the most frequent) alcohol-involved injuries, such as minor cuts, bruises, or burns, do not require medical attention. These events thus do not come to the attention of medical institutions and can be identified only via self reports. It would be nearly impossible to obtain accurate BAC data for such events. The most severe non-fatal alcohol-involved injuries are most likely to be treated in a hospital emergency room or a specialized trauma center. Depending on the facility's protocol, the BAC of all patients or selected patients may be measured in the course of preparation for treatment. Emergency rooms typically measure BAC only in selected patients, as deemed necessary by medical staff. Between these extremes of severity are non-life-threatening injuries for which medical care is sought from a physician or clinic on an outpatient basis or at a hospital (usually at the emergency room). Physicians and outpatient clinics rarely measure BAC.

As discussed in Chapter 6, a risk of alcohol-involved traffic crashes is associated with the distribution of drivers' BAC. Most traffic crashes involve damage only to the vehicle(s) involved, and property-damage outcomes are handled within the Legal Sanctions Subsystem. However, alcohol-involved traffic crashes are more likely than non-alcohol-involved crashes to result in injury or death of drivers, passengers, or pedestrians. Nighttime crashes are more likely than daytime crashes to involve a drinking driver and are more severe than daytime crashes, resulting in more injuries (Rosenberg, Laessig & Rawlings, 1974). These injuries and deaths stimulate a response from the Social, Economic, and Health Consequences Subsystem.

The annual number of drinking and driving injuries and fatalities can be estimated by the general method shown in Fig. 7.5; however, the probability of driving must be taken into account as well. Using four consumption classes ($i = 1$ to 4), the general distribution of the incidence of traffic outcomes by BAC level for a given BAC range (j) can be expressed as:

$$\text{Traffic Outcome (BAC range } j) = (\text{Events}_{1j} \times \text{RR}_{1j}) + (\text{Events}_{2j} \times \text{RR}_{2j}) + (\text{Events}_{3j} \times \text{RR}_{3j}) + (\text{Events}_{4j} \times \text{RR}_{4j})$$

where Events_{ij} = driving events in BAC range j for consumption class i, and RR_{ij} = relative risk of this outcome for consumption class i with a driving event in BAC range j.

The relative risk term above can be further decomposed into at least two terms:

$$\text{RR}_{ij} = \text{DR}_{ij} \times \text{GR}_j$$

where DR_{ij} = the differential relative risk of a crash for consumption class i in BAC range j, and GR_j = the general risk of a crash in BAC range j. These two terms reflect, respectively, the influence of a given level of drinking experience on the risk of a traffic crash associated with a specific BAC range, and the general risk of a traffic crash associated with a specific BAC range, independent of consumption class.

Transition from ignoring, to identifying, to community response

In general, unless an alcohol-involved event or process is disruptive to the community in some way, it may be ignored by the community system (e.g., having hangovers at home is not likely to be identified as a problem). When the event or process becomes disturbing or disruptive (e.g., having hangovers at work), it may be identified as a problem. Immediately or eventually, a community response will be developed, which may create or increase demand for health and social services within the community system. Responses may be developed to address the problem's immediate effects or consequences, or to prevent future occurrences. Alcohol-involved problems may be addressed within existing general health and social services, or through specialized services for alcoholism and alcohol dependency.

One illustration of a dynamic community response is action towards public intoxication. Some 200 years ago in most industrialized societies, public drunkenness might not have been a major community problem and might even have been accepted, tolerated, or expected. In some non-industrialized cultures today, drunkenness in response to the death of a family member may be expected and encouraged; in such cultures, failure to become intoxicated following a family death would violate a norm and could conceivably be identified as a "problem." In recent decades in industrialized societies, public drunkenness was increasingly defined as a community problem, and legal or social responses were developed. A common response through the Legal Sanctions Subsystem was to arrest and jail "public drunks" or remove them from the community by institutionalizing them (see Cook et al., 1973). Many communities also developed non-legal, social responses to this problem, through private agencies such as rescue missions or through hospitals that provided short-term, emergency care. Over time, public health and law enforcement officials learned that legal-system responses to public inebriates (arrest and incarceration) resulted in high recidivism rates; legal-system responses were expensive and did not re-establish inebriates as productive members of the community. To reduce costs and increase benefits to the community, public decision-makers began to develop alternative approaches emphasizing rehabilitation.

Community services that respond to alcohol problems

In response to alcohol-involved problems, as well as other health and social problems, the Social, Economic, and Health Consequences Subsystem typically provides health and medical care services, alcohol dependency services, social services, employment services, and workplace services.

Health and medical care for the consequences of alcohol use can include both general medical care required because of chronic drinking, and acute medical care required because of the acute physical consequences of high-volume drinking at a particular moment or impairment contributing to injury. *General medical care* can include both outpatient and inpatient treatment required for such alcohol-related medical problems as cirrhosis of the liver, alcohol gastritis, intestinal problems (including cancer), and throat cancer. Such treatment is intended to reduce the threat to life as a result of long-term drinking and to improve physical health. *Acute medical care* includes treatment for injuries resulting from impairment of the patient or of someone else (such as a drinking driver or an intoxicated assailant). It also includes treatment for alcohol poisoning and for withdrawal from alcohol (delirium tremens, or DTs). Acute medical care services are provided in emergency rooms, trauma centers, and inpatient facilities and, if the injury is not severe, by private physicians and general health clinics.

Alcohol dependency services are specialized services that assist the alcohol-dependent or alcohol-abusing patient or client in recovery. The long-term objective (often not achieved) is to prevent future heavy drinking events (or at least reduce their frequency) or for patients or clients to maintain abstinence. Services of this type can be provided in a wide range of settings and institutions, and by a variety of providers; a number of treatment and recovery modalities exist. (See Hester & Miller, 1989, for a discussion of the scientific evidence for the effectiveness of various treatment modalities.)

The self-help group Alcoholics Anonymous is a support service for alcohol-dependent persons available in most communities. Al-Anon provides support for family members (usually spouses), and Al-Ateen provides support for young people with alcohol-dependent parents. (See Mäkelä, 1991; and McCrady & Miller, 1993, for a discussion of Alcoholics Anonymous and other self-help societies.) Self-help groups afford opportunities for volunteers (who may or may not be dependent themselves) to assist in the recovery process of alcohol-dependent persons. Self-help groups and volunteers could be viewed as natural (not formally planned or managed) community system responses to problem drinkers.

Formal inpatient and medically supervised residential alcoholism treatment services are provided by general and psychiatric hospitals, and accredited alcoholism treatment units or institutions. Organized non-medically supervised alcoholism treatment programs are provided in residential centers. Social living settings (halfway houses) provide social support for recovery and may or may not have formal treatment programs. Non-residential alcoholism treatment or recovery services also are provided through hospitals or certified residential facilities. Ambulatory outpatient treatment can be provided by medical (psychiatric), psychological, social work, or other licensed professionals or, in some communities, by non-licensed counselors. Both inpatient and outpatient treatment or recovery services may be provided individually or to groups. (See review of alcoholism treatment responses in 16 countries by Klingemann, Takala & Hunt, 1992.)

Social services include services provided by the community in response to non-medical or non-health-related problems that result from drinking. These can include, for example, financial aid to dependent children abandoned by the father as a result of his drinking, or social-service responses to family disruption or violence, such as child or spouse abuse by a drinking family member.

Employment services provide assistance in securing employment, including assistance to people who have lost previous jobs as a result of drinking. *Workplace services* are provided by an employer to assist employees with drinking problems. Often called Employee Assistance Programs (EAPs), such services are designed to identify employees with drinking problems, help them to enter some form of alcohol-dependence recovery program, and help them to maintain their employment while seeking recovery. EAP services often identify problem-drinking employees and refer them to specialized treatment services.

Figure 7.6 illustrates some of the pathways by which alcohol-involved problems create demand for health and social services, and stimulate health and social services responses within the Social, Economic, and Health Consequences Subsystem.

For example, employees with drinking problems (perhaps manifested in work problems such as absenteeism, workplace accidents, or lowered work performance) can be identified by an EAP, resulting in referrals (and thus demand) for alcoholism treatment services. Alternately, alcohol-dependent

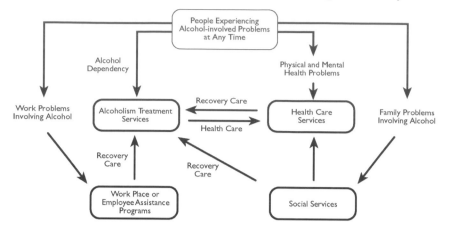

Figure 7.6 Social and health services as a part of the Social, Economic, and Health Consequences Subsystem.

individuals may be referred to alcoholism treatment services by their families, friends, or physicians, or they may refer themselves. Health problems associated with long-term drinking and trauma from alcohol-involved accidents or traffic crashes create demand for medical care. Patients receiving general or acute medical care may subsequently enter alcoholism treatment services to facilitate recovery. Family problems, such as family violence, can come to the attention of social workers (or health-care workers), creating demand for social services to the families and recovery care for the family members with drinking problems.

Economic consequences of alcohol problems

The Social, Economic, and Health Consequences Subsystem incurs economic costs as a result of alcohol-involved problems both directly, in providing the services, and indirectly, through other economic losses resulting from alcohol-involved problems.

The subsystem consumes public and private economic resources directly in providing social and health services in response to problems in which alcohol is a causal factor (whether sole or contributing). Examples are the cost of emergency services to victims in a drinking and driving crash, hospital inpatient services for alcoholics or other heavy drinkers whose physical (or emotional) health has been damaged by long-term drinking, and social services in response to family violence or disruptions involving drinking. These resources can be provided either from public (governmental) sources (e.g., national, state, or local taxes) or from private sources, such as insurance companies, individual income or personal funds, philanthropic organizations, or private companies on behalf of their employees (or members of employees' families).

Direct costs of services are expressed in the budgets of care-giving agencies or in the unit cost for services (e.g., an inpatient hospital day) charged or billed to an individual or an institution, such as an employer or insurance company. Costs for services are a convenient metric with which to establish the relative cost of alcohol-involved problems to the community system, in terms of economic resources consumed by the Social, Economic, and Health Consequences Subsystem. (For discussion of the economic costs of alcohol-involved problems, see Heien & Pittman, 1989; Rice, Kelman & Miller, 1990; and Godfrey, 1991.)

Measurements of direct costs of services also have been used to assess costs for alcoholism treatment. See Holder (1987), Holder & Blose (1992), and Holder et al. (1991). See Hallan & Holder (1986) for an example of computer simulation to estimate the total costs for treatment in a population of alcoholics using various mixes of treatment services.

A second source of costs to the community are related social costs, or what economists sometimes call "opportunity" costs. Such costs include economic loss to employers resulting from reduced productivity by drinking employees and loss of wages (and thus of tax revenues) resulting from alcohol-related absenteeism, injuries, or death. They also include loss of family economic support resulting from drinking, which lowers family standards of living, increases the risk of family instability, and may result in increased delinquency among children. These indirect costs can be used in establishing a public accounting of the losses to the total community system as a result of alcohol-involved problems (For discussion of social costs related to drinking, see Rice, Kelman & Miller 1990; Miller et al., 1995; and Godfrey & Maynard, 1995.)

Interactions with other subsystems

The Social, Economic, and Health Consequences Subsystem identifies and responds to alcohol-involved problems within the community system. This subsystem functions as a safety net in providing health and social services to people who experience problems as a result of their drinking or the drinking of others. Figure 7.7 illustrates interactions of the Social, Economic, and Health Consequences Subsystem with the Consumption, Legal Sanctions, and Social Norms Subsystems.

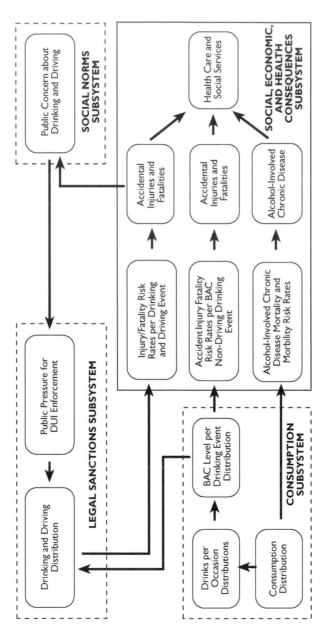

Figure 7.7 Interaction between the Social, Economic and Health Consequences Subsystem and the Social Norms, Legal Sanctions, and Consumption Subsystems.

The most straightforward relationship is between the distributions of alcohol consumption (within the Consumption Subsystem) and the rates of alcohol-involved outcomes in the Social, Economic, and Health Consequences Subsystem. People who consume alcohol at high levels over long periods have much higher individual risks of alcohol-involved chronic disease morbidity and mortality than do drinkers whose average consumption is lower. Thus, as illustrated at the bottom of Fig. 7.7, the distribution of consumption produces associated rates of alcohol-involved chronic diseases. Such diseases create demand for medical services within the Social, Economic, and Health Consequences Subsystem. Similarly, the distribution of DPO (within the Consumption Subsystem) produces a distribution of BAC; high volumes of consumption per occasion (regardless of overall average consumption), expressed as high BACs, are associated with increased risk of alcohol-involved injuries and fatalities. Such events also contribute to community demand for medical services.

The input from the Consumption Subsystem to the Social, Economic, and Health Consequences Subsystem with respect to non-traffic injuries and fatalities is shown in the middle of Fig. 7.7. When drinking and driving is involved, the interaction of DPO (from the Consumption Subsystem) with driving patterns (in the Legal Sanctions Subsystem) determines the rate of alcohol-involved traffic injuries and fatalities, as illustrated at the top of Fig. 7.7.

In turn, the Social, Economic, and Health Consequences Subsystem provides input to the Social Norms Subsystem. As discussed in Chapter 5, drinking norms are influenced by community concern about alcohol-involved problems, which in turn is affected by public awareness of the social, economic, and health consequences of alcohol use.

8

Community-level alcohol problem prevention

Introduction

The goal of prevention is to reduce the future occurrence of alcohol-involved problems, which (as defined in this book) are the natural products (output) of the community system. How to develop effective long-term interventions or changes in this complex, open, and adaptive system is neither simple nor obvious. As an adaptive system, the community will not be affected by prevention programs or efforts that make no changes in the system's structure or processes. Furthermore, the system will adjust to and compensate for prevention efforts that do alter its natural arrangements. Such community system adjustments hamper the potential long-term effectiveness of any prevention intervention and are the most serious obstacle to cost-effective alcohol problem prevention in the long term.

For example, consider what happens in the community if enforcement against drinking and driving is increased, and, as a result of publicity about increased enforcement, drivers believe their chance of being detected and arrested for driving under the influence (DUI) is now much higher (i.e., perceived risk of arrest increases). If the actual risk of arrest has increased only slightly (so that it is much lower than the new perceived risk), then, over time, drivers will learn that their perceived risk is much too high. As a result, they will naturally return to their prior drinking and driving behavior, and little or no long-term reduction in alcohol-involved crashes will result. Similarly, consider the effects of increasing the retail prices of alcoholic beverages, say by 10%. Although some drinkers may reduce their alcohol consumption, many can maintain it at the initial level by purchasing less-expensive brands or substituting beverage types (e.g., beer or wine for spirits). As another example, consider the effects of training teenagers at school about the harm of drinking. If alcohol remains readily available to teens at retail stores and at social gatherings, then teen drinking is unlikely to be changed, and education is likely to have at best a transient effect on the drinking patterns of that cohort. In each of these scenarios, the community system naturally adjusts to purposeful efforts to reduce alcohol use and alcohol problems.

This chapter first reviews potential approaches to identifying intervention points and alcohol problem prevention strategies within the community system, using alcohol-involved traffic crashes and non-traffic injuries as examples. Ways in which prevention programs and policies can be selected in order to affect such intervention points (i.e., actually make changes in the system) are presented. Potential system effects then are illustrated through the use of the computer model *SimCom*, to project future trends in one outcome variable – driver fatalities – and to compare the projected long-term effects of alternative interventions. Finally, the implications of a systems perspective for community alcohol problem prevention are discussed.

Interventions to prevent alcohol-involved problems in a complex community system

Any prevention program, policy, or strategy, whatever its content or design, can potentially disrupt, transform, or change a community system. However, most contemporary prevention programs, making no system changes, have, in the end, little actual effect on alcohol problems. Even if such programs have the potential to affect a specific target group within the drinking population, self-adaptive community systems, by their very nature, adjust to prevention efforts and mitigate their long-term effects.

Alcohol problem prevention interventions are actions, activities, efforts, or policies intended to reduce the future occurrence of alcohol-involved problems. Interventions to reduce alcohol-involved problems rarely affect the problems directly; rather, they most often affect intermediate variables (factors that influence the risk or potential of problems), which in turn affect the problems directly. This causal chain is illustrated by Fig. 8.1, in which the alcohol-involved problem is caused by three intermediate variables, X, Y, and Z. Four possible prevention interventions are identified that have the potential to change one or more of the intermediate variables. For example, intervention B is capable of affecting intermediate variables X and Y, while intervention A can affect only variable X.

Figure 8.2 illustrates intermediate variables and interventions that affect the outcome variable of alcohol-involved traffic crashes. The occurrence of alcohol-involved crashes is related to the number of driving events (over a

Interventions   Intermediate   Target
                        Variables   Outcome

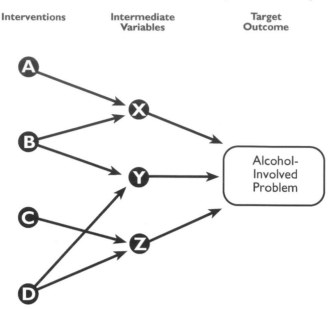

Figure 8.1 Causal chain: relationship of prevention interventions to intermediate
variables to a target outcome.

defined period of time) in which the drivers have been drinking. BAC is an
indicator of the driver's level of impairment from alcohol. Therefore, an
important intermediate variable is the number of driving trips over a given
period (e.g., one month or one year) in which the drivers have any non-zero
BAC or have a high BAC (e.g., over 0.05%). This intermediate variable can
be represented as a distribution of the number of driving trips by ranges of
drivers' BACs. Of course, most driving events involving alcohol do not
result in crashes. The overall risk of alcohol-involved crashes results from
the interaction of the general risk of a crash with the increased risk
associated with driver impairment from alcohol. Because, on average, the
risk of an alcohol-involved crash increases with increased BAC, driving
events at higher driver BACs carry, on average, greater individual risks of
crashes. Thus, another intermediate variable is the distribution of crash
risk by driver BAC. The interaction of these two intermediate variables at
specific BAC values produces the distribution of traffic crashes by driver
BAC, which can be summed as the total traffic crashes within the community over a given period. The alcohol-involved traffic crashes are those in
which the drivers had non-zero BACs. See discussion in Chapter 6.

   A prevention strategy that increases DUI enforcement can affect the

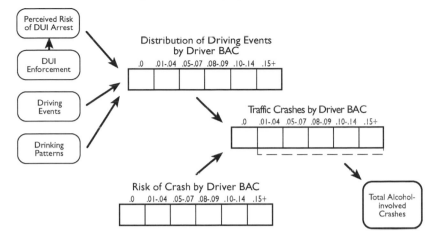

Figure 8.2 Intermediate variables and interventions for alcohol-involved traffic crashes.

distribution of alcohol-involved driving events. Increased DUI enforcement does not reduce the risk of a crash associated with any individual alcohol-involved driving event. Rather, it can alter the distribution of alcohol-involved driving events to increase the number of zero- to low-BAC driving events relative to the number of high-BAC driving events. This change in distribution in turn reduces the overall risk of alcohol-involved crashes. Thus, enforcement does not affect crashes directly, but affects an intermediate variable – the distribution of driving events involving alcohol, which in turn affects the risk of crashes.

The distribution of driving events by driver BAC and the distribution of crash risk by BAC are in turn influenced by other intermediate variables that can be changed by prevention interventions. For example, the distribution of driving events by driver BAC can be influenced by drivers' perceptions of their risk of DUI arrest (as discussed in Chapter 6). Thus, both the perceived risk of arrest and the actual DUI enforcement level can potentially change the distribution of driving events by driver BAC, which in turn can change the frequency of alcohol-involved crashes. Of course, the total amount of driving (numbers and distances of trips) affects the risk of crashes, regardless of whether drivers have been drinking. Changes in the total number of trips can also affect the distribution of driving events by driver BAC. A gasoline shortage or a substantial increase in gasoline prices could reduce the number of trips made over a given period and thus

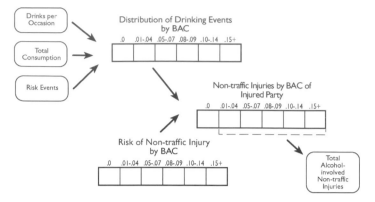

Figure 8.3 Intermediate variables and interventions for alcohol-involved non-traffic injuries.

could reduce the number of driving events in which the driver had been drinking.

Each of the intermediate variables identified in this example is a candidate target for preventive intervention to reduce the final alcohol-involved outcome variable, alcohol-involved traffic crashes. Although it is unlikely that a gasoline shortage would purposely be created in order to reduce alcohol-involved traffic crashes, a safety (and fiscal) policy to increase gasoline excise taxes in order to reduce driving events could also have the effect of reducing alcohol-involved traffic crashes. Certainly, increasing the level of DUI enforcement or increasing drivers' perceived risk of detection by law enforcement are potential preventive interventions. Other interventions might be designed to lower the risk of crashes in general or the risk of crashes as a function of BAC level. Improvements in roadways or lowering of the speed limit are examples of changes that lower the risk of crashes in general and thus lower the risk of alcohol-involved crashes.

Figure 8.3 further illustrates the causal chain linking prevention interventions with intermediate variables that affect an alcohol-involved problem. In this example, the problem is alcohol-involved non-traffic injuries (e.g., burns, falls, swimming accidents, cuts, and assaults occurring in conjunction with alcohol use). As with traffic crashes, many non-traffic injuries have no alcohol involvement; however, drinking generally increases the risk of each type of injury. In other words, as BAC increases, one's risk of a non-traffic injury also increases.

In Fig. 8.3, one intermediate variable is the risk of injury as a function of BAC – the distribution that reflects the increased risk or probability of an injury with increasing BAC. (The first category in this distribution represents the base risk of injury if a person has not been drinking (BAC = 0.0).) Another key intermediate variable is the pattern of drinking. The amount of alcohol consumed during a drinking occasion establishes the level of impairment resulting from alcohol use (represented in Fig. 8.3 as the distribution of drinking events by BAC). If this drinking is done in conjunction with an activity involving risk of injury, then an alcohol-involved non-traffic injury can result. The interaction of two intermediate variables – the distribution of drinking events by BAC and the distribution of risk of injury by BAC – produces the distribution of non-traffic injuries by BAC.

One approach to preventing injuries is to reduce people's participation in risky activities, such as climbing stairs or ladders, engaging in water activities, or smoking in bed. Another approach is to reduce the average number of drinks consumed during a drinking event; lowering the number of drinks per occasion will result in lowered BAC (level of impairment) and thus lowered risk of injury. Changes in overall average personal alcohol consumption can also affect the distribution of drinks per occasion or BAC (level of impairment), thus affecting the risk of injury.

Relationships of interventions to effects on intermediate variables

Alcohol problem prevention interventions (programs or policies) are effective primarily by changing intermediate variables, which in turn affect alcohol-involved problems or outcomes. Prevention interventions can be characterized along a continuum of strength or extent; any type of intervention may vary in strength as a result of many factors of implementation and public acceptance. The strength of an intervention typically is described as its "dosage," a term derived with reference to prescription drugs in clinical preventive or treatment trials. Here, "dosage" is used to refer to the extent, size, strength, and duration of a prevention program or policy.

Extending the prescription drug analogy, an intervention's "dose-response relationship" can be described as the changes in an intermediate variable that are expected to result from given "dosages" of an intervention. For example, using the traffic-crash illustration from Fig. 8.2 (above), one could consider the relationship between the dosage of an intervention (e.g., a mass-media campaign about DUI enforcement) and the level of perceived risk of DUI arrest. In other words, one could determine the dose-response relationship between mass communications initiatives and changes in perceived risk of DUI arrest.

One possible dose-response relationship is illustrated in Fig. 8.4. Here, the dose response is characterized as linear; that is, for each incremental

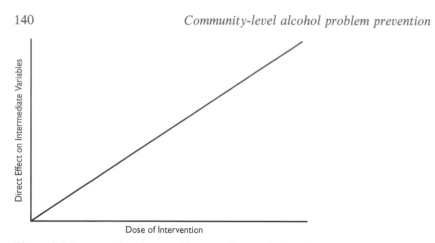

Figure 8.4 Intervention dose and intermediate variable effect – straight line.

increase in dosage, there is a corresponding direct incremental increase in the intervention's effect on the intermediate variable, resulting in a straight-line dose-response curve. This relationship has often been assumed in many alcohol problem prevention programs.

In practice, non-linear dose-response relationships also are possible, as illustrated in Fig. 8.5. In this example, curve A illustrates what could be called a "barrier" relationship between intervention dosage and effect: beyond a certain dosage, the net increase in effect per unit increase in intervention dosage is quite small. Curve B illustrates what could be called a "threshold" relationship: incremental increases in intervention dosage produce very small, if any, increases in effect until a certain dosage is reached; however, starting at that threshold dosage, each incremental increase in dosage produces a greater increase in effect, resulting in an exponential dose-response curve. Curve C illustrates yet a third possible non-linear dose-response relationship, which could be called a "step" relationship: unit increases in intervention dosage produce only small changes in the intermediate variable until a certain dosage is reached that produces a major effect (as in the threshold relationship). However, further increases in intervention dosage produce no further change in the inter-mediate variable, resulting in an S-shaped dose-response curve.

The four possible relationships between intervention dosage and the expected effect on an intermediate variable shown in Figs. 8.4 and 8.5 represent but a few of the possible real-world relationships. In practice, the dose-response relationship of a prevention intervention is seldom obvious or easily predictable.

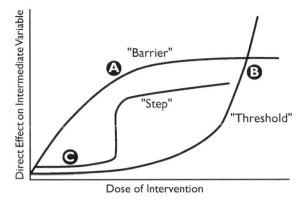

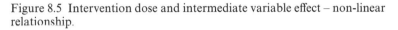

Figure 8.5 Intervention dose and intermediate variable effect – non-linear relationship.

Prevention within a community system

The past 20 years have seen a virtual explosion of research on the risk factors for alcohol-involved problems and the potential effectiveness of various strategies or approaches to alcohol problem prevention (e.g., see Edwards et al., 1994, for a review of research on the effectiveness of alcohol policy in prevention). However, little or no use of such scientific evidence has been made in the design or evaluation of most community prevention programs for alcohol or other drug abuse. Current practice lags well behind the state of scientific knowledge about alcohol-involved problems, and current understanding of the implications of this knowledge for prevention program design and planning. As a result, most current prevention programs at the community level are unlikely to yield the results desired by their designers and implementors. See discussion by Holder (1992).

A community systems approach to alcohol problem prevention, as presented here, establishes two important demands on the prevention planner. First, the planner must understand that system changes (possible interventions) with real potential to reduce alcohol problems are not "discovered" through prevention programs; they are identified and understood via scientific study. Second, the planner must appreciate and understand the complexity of the community system sufficiently to identify those points at which interventions have real potential to reduce future problems. To have a chance at real reduction of future alcohol-involved problems, prevention programs must make the best use of available scientific evidence in their design.

Community-level alcohol information programs, based on the catchment-area perspective, have been tried frequently in the past and are quite popular at present. They typically entail investments in education and public awareness, reflecting the belief (or hope) that a "shot" of prevention will render the community safe. Increased knowledge or awareness does not in itself change drinking patterns, alcohol availability, community norms about drinking, or the role of alcohol in routine community activities or processes. Most such educational programs have had little long-term impact on drinking behavior; their effect largely has been limited to increasing the amount of information people have about alcohol and altering their attitudes, without affecting their behaviors. (For reviews of evidence on the effectiveness of school and public education, see Blane & Hewitt, 1977; Cameron, 1979; Moskowitz, 1989; and Casswell, 1995.)

Further complicating the challenge of alcohol problem prevention is the reality that within health-conscious communities, drinking alcohol is not as unambivalently considered to constitute a health risk as, say, eating butter or red meat; in the latter cases, abstinence or highly controlled use are popular consumer options. Similarly, facts about the health risks of alcohol use and social norms against drinking do not have as great an impact as those concerning smoking, where in recent years problem prevention has emphasized abstinence rather than moderation. Moderate use of alcohol is socially accepted, and personal abstinence is not always a preferred social or epidemiological prevention goal except for alcoholics.

A long tradition exists of alcohol problem prevention through public policy (government control and regulation of alcoholic beverages). In most industrialized societies there is some form of agency, department, bureau, or organization for alcoholic beverage control, which regulates the licensing of establishments to sell alcohol for on-premises or off-premises consumption. In addition, legally unacceptable levels of alcohol in the bloodstream (BAC) have been established for operators of motor vehicles (i.e., *per se* limits at which a person is legally considered too impaired to drive). Lower limits are set for drivers of commercial vehicles, and airline pilots are not allowed to fly with any non-zero BAC. In targeting whole populations rather than problem drinkers, such policies reflect a systems perspective.

The most successful prevention strategies to date have employed public policies that affect access to alcohol. A recent example is the raising of the minimum alcohol purchase age to 21 in all states of the US. This restriction of access to alcohol has been shown to reduce alcohol-involved traffic crashes among 18- to 20-year-olds. (For discussion of research on minimum drinking age, see Wagenaar, 1983; the US General Accounting Office, 1987; and O'Malley & Wagenaar, 1991.) Another system strategy that has been considered (but not often implemented) for reducing alcohol-involved traffic crashes and cirrhosis mortality is to use the price sensitivity of alcohol purchases to reduce access to alcohol (see Cook & Tauchen, 1982, in the US; and Godfrey, 1990, in Great Britain). See review of international research on price by Österberg (1995). Recent evidence suggests that public information via the news media can increase acceptance of and support for local public policy approaches to alcohol problem prevention (Casswell, 1995). Hence, prevention strategies that couple community structural changes affecting alcohol access, law enforcement, and server training with well-planned and intensive media efforts have a real potential for success (for further discussion, see Hochheimer, 1981; and Holder & Blose, 1983). See Holder (1993) and Holder et al. (1997/in press) for a discussion, and the results from a multi-component community prevention trial developed to make structural changes.

The role of computer-based models of the community system

An appreciative awareness of the community as a complex adaptive system, as described in previous chapters, is not sufficient for design and implementation of effective alcohol problem prevention strategies. It simply is not possible for a prevention practitioner to simultaneously consider all the community subsystems and determine the potential future effects of prevention interventions within the community system. To deal with the complexity of the community system, the prevention planner needs assistance. A promising form of technological assistance in prevention planning as described in Chapter 1 is the use of computer based simulation models that incorporate the natural complexity of community systems.

A specific illustration of the use of computer models to examine the potential effects of alternative prevention strategies, as a practical aid to selection of cost-effective prevention elements, is provided by *SimCom*. This computer model is based upon a complex adaptive systems perspective that captures the principal subsystems of the community system considered necessary for an understanding of alcohol use and alcohol problems, as described in this book. The structure of *SimCom* is mathematically specified and programmed into a computer. Because *SimCom* is not based upon one specific community, it is sufficiently general to apply to any community and sufficiently robust to be loaded with local data to capture the uniqueness of specific communities. This ability to generalize increases scientific confidence in the model, as well as its practical utility. The purpose of *SimCom* is both to advance the science of alcohol problem prevention and to provide a practical tool to assist prevention planners. The development and scientific testing of *SimCom* are described elsewhere (Holder & Blose, 1983, 1987, 1988; Holder, 1996*a*).

SimCom is a causal model, designed to simulate a real community when loaded with appropriate local data. It also can be used for simulations at a national or regional level. *SimCom* differs in two critical ways from the vast majority of computer modeling applications for community-level policy and planning in general, and for alcohol problem prevention research in particular. First, a single, general model structure has been developed to capture the principal dynamics of a community system with respect to alcohol use. This structure is sufficiently general to apply to any community, yet sufficiently detailed to capture the uniqueness of specific communities through initial data loadings. One criticism of the application of computer modeling to urban land use and transportation planning in the 1970s was that planners in various local jurisdictions, who were trying to deal with the same conceptual and methodological issues, were building an essentially unique model for each jurisdiction (Kain, 1978). A more recent criticism of planning tools with presumed universal applicability is that they are too general, being based on data structures (e.g., spreadsheet layouts) rather than on problem content (Klosterman, 1986; also see Rydell & Everingham, 1994, for an example of such a spreadsheet model for illicit drug prevention). The approach used here has the virtue of not requiring communities to start from scratch for each local application, while remaining rich in research-based understanding of community behaviors and dynamics.

A second difference between *SimCom* and most other computer-based policy applications is the model's anticipated role in the prevention planning process. In most applications, models are used only to evaluate specific policies predefined by planners and policy-makers. In contrast, *SimCom* is a tool to assist the community in understanding the complex factors involved in alcohol use and alcohol-involved problems, and to support the planning process itself. This model also is an intellectual vehicle for accumulating and synthesizing the best available research in the field; in a sense, it serves as an evolving research platform and theory-building mechanism.

The first-generation *SimCom* model, begun in 1980, permitted a test of the general approach to causal modeling of a community with regard to its alcohol use (Holder & Blose, 1983). The model was validated at the national level and initially tested at the local level in three US communities (Alameda County, California; Washington County, Vermont; and Wake County, North Carolina). Development of the second-generation model focused on validation of two subsystems, alcohol consumption, and drinking and driving, in a targeted community (San Diego County, California), and subsequently was used to test a range of interventions (Holder & Blose, 1987, 1988). Development of the third-generation model focused again on San Diego County. Fourth- and fifth-generation models have focused on tests in ten US states and 20 communities. (See Holder, 1996*b*, for a description of the application of computer simulation to analyzing the possible effects of local alcohol policy in the community.)

To use *SimCom* in planning, one must:

(1) Identify the alcohol-involved problem(s) one wishes to reduce.
(2) Specify the intermediate variable(s) in which changes could potentially reduce these problems.
(3) Make within *SimCom* the changes in the intermediate variable(s) that specific alcohol-prevention policies or programs are anticipated to achieve.

In other words, the prevention designer must know, from existing scientific evidence or professional experience, which intermediate variable(s) the prevention strategies will affect and the anticipated sizes of such effects on key intermediate variables.

The *SimCom* model recreates the systems dynamics of a targeted community with regard to alcohol retail activity, alcohol consumption patterns, drinking and driving behavior, social norms, and regulatory controls. Published research findings, survey data, and results from secondary data analyses are used to define and mathematically specify relationships among variables within and across the model subsystems. Annual outcomes generated by the model include the distribution of alcohol consumption by age and gender groups, alcohol retail sales, new licenses for on-premises and off-premises sale of alcoholic beverages, DUI arrests and convictions, driver fatalities, crashes resulting in injury, and measures of mortality, morbidity, and the socioeconomic consequences of problem drinking. The types of data used for calibrating and testing the model are illustrated in Table 8.1.

Once the model's congruence with historical data has been established, a series of potential prevention interventions can be proposed and their likely effects on alcohol-involved problems simulated over, say, a ten-year period. The general procedure is to:

Table 8.1. *Selected variables for benchmark and prevention strategy testing*

Subsystem	Model variables	System measures	Data sources
Consumption	Alcohol sales	Annual retail sales by beverage	Dept. of Revenue or Taxation
	Age–sex consumption	Local consumption by beverage by age and sex group	Local, state, or national alcohol consumption surveys
Retail sales	Retail businesses	Local retail outlets	State, local, or national business surveys
	Alcohol sale permits	License counts	Alcohol Beverage Control Dept.
Legal sanctions	Driver fatalities	Annual number of fatalities	Dept. of Transportation
	Injury crashes	Annual number of crashes	Dept. of Transportation
	Alcohol-related arrests/ convictions	DUI, underage sales, public intoxication	Local law enforcement/criminal justice statistics
Social norms	Public awareness	Local news coverage	Newspaper content analysis
	Public concern	Concern about alcohol problems	Local surveys
Social, economic, and health consequences	Non-traffic injuries	Annual number of non-traffic injuries	Dept. of Health
	Alcohol-related deaths	Alcohol mortality for selected ICD codes	Dept. of Health
	Alcoholism treatment	Annual admissions to treatment	Alcohol Authority or Health Services
	Alcohol-related family violence	Child abuse/neglect with alcohol involvement	Dept. of Social Services or Welfare

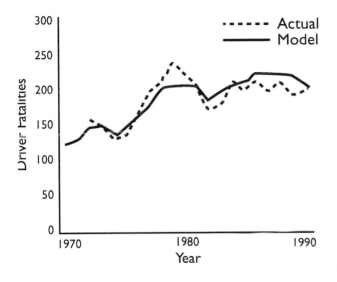

Figure 8.6 Benchmark results for driver fatality estimates vs. actual in San Diego, California (USA)

(1) Establish a congruent model.
(2) Use the model to alter intermediate variables.
(3) Run the model with and without these changes.
(4) Compare the long-term levels of alcohol problems predicted with and without the proposed system changes.

Alternative prevention strategies can be compared by running the model with different values for selected policy variables. Where possible, the model's forecasting capability should be evaluated by contrasting its predictions against results actually obtained when similar policy variables were changed in other communities. Where the proposed policy change has never previously been implemented, model forecasts may be compared with the most closely relevant research findings. Once a model is validated for a particular community, community groups can use it to investigate the anticipated impacts of potentially costly interventions before introducing them.

For a complete description of *SimCom* and to inquire about participating in further field testing of this model, contact the author of this book at the Prevention Research Center, 2150 Shattuck Avenue, Suite 900, Berkeley, CA 94704 (USA).

Benchmark testing of the model

The first step in testing a computer model is to test its ability to recreate history (which actually tests the model builder's understanding of the real system). Because *SimCom* is a causal, mathematical model of alcohol use and alcohol problems, only the initial loading values are used in this benchmark testing (e.g., values for the year 1970). The model is started, and interactions between and among the internal variables determine the key outcome data. (In such a causal model, no curve-fitting is used.)

Benchmark testing of *SimCom* for San Diego, California, is illustrated in Fig. 8.6. In this example, driver fatalities are the outcome variable; in the US, 40 to 50% of these deaths are alcohol-involved (as discussed in Chapter 6). The figure plots the actual fatality count and the model simulation result over the period 1970 to 1990. Obviously, the model cannot re-create history perfectly, but, as this illustration shows, it matches well the major trends in this variable over the period of simulation. Thus, the model can be used to provide a reasonable projection of future trends.

Using the model to project the results of prevention interventions

Because the *SimCom* model can be used to predict future trends in alcohol-involved outcome variables (e.g., driver fatalities), it can also be used to test the potential effects of prevention interventions on such outcomes (e.g., to test whether a planned intervention can reduce driver fatalities from the number otherwise expected over a given period). Because not all driver fatalities involve drinking, only the portion involving alcohol will be affected by alcohol-specific prevention strategies. *SimCom* can be used to examine the potential effects of other future events on the outcome variables, as well. For example, a future gasoline shortage could result in a major increase in gasoline prices, which would be likely to lower the total frequency of driving, the total number of crashes, and thus the number of alcohol-involved crashes. *SimCom* could also be used to project the effects of such an event.

The major intermediate variables that affect alcohol-involved driver fatalities are described in Chapter 6. Figure 8.7 summarizes how the key factors related to drinking and driving interact to affect this outcome variable. Examination of Fig. 8.7 also suggests potential intervention points for prevention. The interaction of the distribution of driving events by driver BAC with the crash risk distribution (which also is related to driver BAC) yields the number of alcohol-related traffic crashes resulting in injury and the number of driver fatalities.

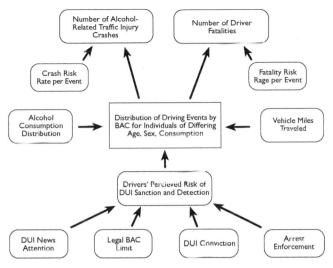

Figure 8.7 Factors relating to drinking and driving which suggest potential prevention interventions.

In general, the dynamics of the distribution of drinking and driving within *SimCom* can be described by the equation:

$$\text{Drink/Drive}_{t+1} = Q \, (\text{Drink/Drive}_t)$$

where Q is a transformational operator that relates changes in such variables as drinks per occasion by consumption class, perceived risk of DUI detection and sanctions, and miles traveled, to changes in the drinking and driving distribution – that is, it transforms the distribution at time t to obtain the distribution at time t + 1. In other words, Q is a function of those intermediate variables:

$$Q = f \, (\text{drinks per occasion by consumption class, perceived risk of DUI detection, driving patterns})$$

Within *SimCom*, the transformational operator Q changes the distribution of driving events by driver BAC by altering the three empirically determined parameters (a, b, and c) of the equation given in Chapter 6.

Candidate intermediate variables for prevention interventions

The following major variables affect the drinking and driving distribution (i.e., the distribution of driving events by driver BAC) over time:

- Changes in the distribution of drinks per occasion (DPO). Because non-zero-BAC driving events are produced by the joint occurrence of drinking events and driving events, changes in DPO will affect the distribution of drinking and driving events.
- Vehicle miles traveled or the number of driving trips. Again, because non-zero-BAC driving events are produced by the joint occurrence of drinking events and driving events, changes in the number and length of driving trips (and thus the overall driving frequency in a community) will affect the distribution of drinking and driving events.
- Changes in perceived risk of arrest for DUI. Perceived risk is defined as the average estimated probability by the population that a drinking driver will be detected by law enforcement. Perceived risk in turn is related to the legal BAC limit, the level of DUI enforcement, the DUI conviction rate, and news attention to (i.e., public awareness of) DUI enforcement.

The retail price of alcohol has been shown to affect the overall alcohol consumption level; as discussed in Chapter 2, changes in alcohol price can alter DPO. Therefore, the price of alcohol is a candidate intermediate variable for prevention intervention in this example.

Perceived risk of DUI detection and sanctions is a key variable in the relationship between drinking and subsequent driving and, therefore, could be targeted as a powerful intermediate variable for prevention intervention. The research literature provides some guidance about the specific effects of changes in perceived risk on drinking and driving behavior. Most studies measure the effects of changes in risk of arrest or sanctions against outcomes, such as fatalities, single-vehicle crashes, or had-been-drinking crashes.

As discussed in Chapter 6, perceived risk of detection and sanction for DUI depends on public attention to DUI enforcement in the community, which is affected by coverage of this issue in the local news media or other public information sources. The amount of media news coverage of DUI enforcement can be used as a measure of public awareness. Any amount of news coverage of DUI enforcement will have some influence on perceived risk; to sustain a given level of perceived risk, some maintenance level of annual news coverage is required.

SimCom simulation example: the projected effects of alternative prevention interventions on driver fatalities in San Diego, California

Figure 8.8 shows the annual numbers of driver fatalities in San Diego projected for the period 1996 to 2005 by *SimCom* under four sets of

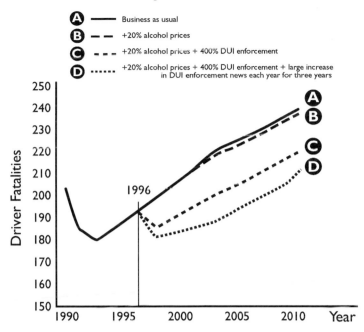

Figure 8.8 Illustration of potential effects on driver fatalities of alternative prevention scenarios in San Diego, California, USA.

conditions. These projections are based on income and population projections developed by the State of California, and assumptions of moderate economic growth during this period. Curve A (the solid line) represents the fatalities projected in the absence of any new alcohol problem prevention interventions during this period – in other words, under conditions of "business as usual." The curve is smooth, reflecting the smooth projections of the key exogenous variables provided by the State. The trend is upward, primarily as a consequence of expected increases in personal income, and economic and population growth.

The first prevention intervention tested in this *SimCom* simulation is a one-time 20% increase in the retail prices of all three types of alcoholic beverage (beer, wine, and spirits) in 1996. This consumption related intervention is projected to result in a very small long-term decrease in driver fatalities, shown as Curve B in Fig. 8.8 (where it is nearly indistinguishable from Curve A). This projected outcome is understandable, in that alcohol is relatively inexpensive in San Diego, where all retail sales of alcohol are through privately owned outlets. The simulation results illustrate the potential of the community system to adjust to this one-time price increase. This adjustment can result from consumers' substituting lower-priced beverages in order to consume the same amount of alcohol at the same cost. This simulation also illustrates that at the local level, a single intervention is unlikely, on its own, to produce dramatic changes in driver fatalities.

The second simulated intervention projects the effects of the same one-time 20% price increase plus a substantial increase in drinking and driving enforcement in 1994 (to five times the current level, for a 400% increase). The projected result of this combined price and enforcement intervention is shown as Curve C in Fig. 8.8. In this simulation, DUI enforcement is increased without any accompanying publicity or purposeful effort to increase public awareness of DUI enforcement via the news media.

The final simulated intervention adds to the one-time price increase and increase in DUI enforcement the following increases in local news coverage of DUI enforcement: a 300% increase in 1996, a 100% increase in 1997, and a 50% increase in 1998. The effect of public exposure to news about DUI enforcement naturally decays over time; therefore, the increase in news coverage each year is designed not only to make up for natural declines in public awareness, but to produce net increases each year over the three years. The projected results of this combined prevention strategy are shown as Curve D in Fig. 8.8.

In general, this illustration shows how a complex systems computer model can be used to investigate one or a combination of potential prevention strategies at the community level. This example also illustrates how a single intervention (in this case, a one-time increase in prices) could have a time-limited effect, as the system adjusts. Even the combined strategy (prices, DUI enforcement, and increased news coverage) does not eliminate all problems or even cause the upward trends in future problems to turn down. Only a net reduction in problem levels is projected. In other words, effective prevention strategies require careful thought and a realistic effectiveness expectation.

Summary

The goal of this book has been to introduce a perspective that views the community as a complex adaptive system and to argue that this perspective is necessary for reducing alcohol-involved problems in the community now and into the 21st century. This book outlines a conceptual model of the community system. This conceptual model also forms the basis of the computer-based model, *SimCom*. While the model is useful as a technical tool to assist community prevention planners, its greatest utility is as a new paradigm of prevention at the community level.

Too frequently, research of value to local decision-makers does not reach them, or they are unable to understand and use it (for discussions of this problem, see Langendorf, 1985, and Giesbrecht, 1993). Furthermore, even when research is valued by community prevention practitioners, it rarely is presented in a way through which it can be applied by local practitioners lacking specialized training. The type of computer simulation model represented by *SimCom* is easier for lay persons to grasp, because the mathematics driving the model is hidden beneath the surface logic, which can be explained to the lay person through easy-to-read flow diagrams.

Application of any computer model developed primarily as a research tool in a community context raises some potential concerns. Such a model may prove to require more data than are feasible to collect in current local prevention practice. Furthermore, the complexity of a sophisticated computer-based model could create a gap between model designers and community practitioners (see discussion by Brewer, 1983; and Holder & Blose, 1988). To what extent do prevention planners need to grasp the full complexity of the model's design? Only to the extent that they wish to have a complete grasp of this complexity in practice. Community practitioners can use the model appropriately even if they are not able to evaluate all the assumptions and interpolations from research and databases outside their community. The availability of a model of their own community with a high degree of historical accuracy gives community prevention practitioners confidence in the model's utility for testing alternative local prevention strategies.

Conclusions – final thoughts from a heretic

If community leaders or prevention planners are unable (or unwilling) to undertake the difficult thinking necessary to improve their understanding of their own community systems, then local prevention interventions selected will have limited (if any) long-term effectiveness. To bring about long-term reduction of alcohol-involved problems, community prevention planners must get involved in some of the same conceptual work and supporting scientific research necessary for a complex adaptive systems perspective, even if they do not use computer modeling technology itself.

A significant paradigm shift occurs when prevention practitioners accept a complex adaptive systems perspective. This perspective has at its core the assumption that alcohol problems result from the complex interactions within the social, economic, and cultural community systems in which people exist. It requires consideration of this larger systems context in which alcohol problems are embedded. For example, even if there were to be a genetic predisposition for some people to become dependent upon alcohol, without alcohol availability in a convenient, affordable form, drinking would be limited.

The major function of a complex system is to survive. All elements of a system are continuously being tested by the system to determine (test, if you will) their contribution to survivability. This suggests that alcohol problems by their very nature contribute in someway to system adaptation and survival. How is this possible? Well, if you take a less dispassionate view of these things, deaths by cirrhosis or highway crashes stimulate medical and police activities, and provide justifications for such subsystems. Where would the police be without crime and traffic crashes? Alcohol-involved injuries and health problems stimulate the medical care sector of the community system, providing a considerable demand for hospital beds, recovery activities, and treatment. Deaths create new opportunities for others, particularly for young people when older people leave the system.

Such observations may be seen by some as cold and uncaring, even inhuman. Actually this view comes closer to recognizing the real functioning of community systems in which alcohol use and abuse occurs than a perspective which only looks at a collection of dysfunctional or disabled drinkers within the community. The selling of alcohol is a major source of money, both for the wholesalers who distribute alcohol, the retailers who sell alcohol, and the taxes which are derived from such sale. There are no incentives for any of these sectors to lower the revenue which alcohol sales produce. Quite the contrary; the economic sector will actively resist efforts which could lower sales. There are many examples of such resistance. The challenge to those who desire to prevent or reduce future alcohol problems at the local level is to become realistic about the community system with which they are confronted.

Once one adopts a complex adaptive system view, then one has a means to understand this system and its behavior. Without a change in perspective, prevention strategies are destined to continue to be ineffective and in many cases irrelevant.

Both researchers and community planners must extend their thinking about prevention and effective countermeasures beyond those that have traditionally been considered. Until systems thinking is a regular part of efforts to reduce alcohol-involved problems, prevention activities will operate in hit-or-miss manner, without substantially reducing the risks of alcohol-involved problems in the community. Until community alcohol problem prevention efforts are based on an appreciation and understanding of the community as a complex adaptive system, they are destined to repeat the mistakes of the past.

In the end, using a community systems perspective for alcohol problem prevention can be quite demanding. The implicit assumption in popular alcohol problem prevention is that heavy and problem drinkers are the core of all alcohol-involved problems; thus, many popular community prevention approaches involve programs that target individuals and groups. However, the systems approach demonstrates that drinking within the total community – including alcohol retail price, alcohol availability, and community values about acceptable and unacceptable drinking – is central to an understanding of alcohol-involved problems and their solutions. Even if target-group approaches succeed in affecting specific individuals (a big "IF," as there is limited evidence that such approaches are effective), a complex adaptive system can and probably will produce replacements for these "fixed-up" individuals if no corresponding structural change is made in the community system.

Furthermore, a systems perspective requires a higher level of knowledge, skills, and planning technology than is currently used by prevention practitioners. For example, to use a computer model such as *SimCom*, the user must at least be able to identify the intermediate variable(s) that are likely to be affected and the size of change in these variables that can realistically be expected from the chosen prevention strategy. This requires a careful analysis of resources available, existing barriers and enabling factors, and evidence of effectiveness of the strategies selected. Personal preference for (or even excitement) about a specific prevention program can not replace careful, high-level prevention planning. Of course, public acceptance of and support for any system intervention are important contributors to successful prevention at the local level.

This book has used complex adaptive systems as a foundation for proposing a systems approach to alcohol use and the prevention of alcohol-involved problems. While the concept of individual adaptation is certainly familiar to alcoholism clinical treatment and research, system adaption is not a major element in prevention practice or research. A true recognition of community system adaptation and its full implication for prevention has been missing.

In the end, a systems approach to prevention of alcohol problems is not simple nor is it easily made operational in practice. The field of alcohol problem prevention stands at a critical junction in its development. To adopt the perspectives proposed in this book is both challenging and rewarding. Some concluding recommendations follow below.

First, the field of alcohol problem prevention should abandon high-risk and target group approaches. This would be painful and difficult for many professionals and advocates in the alcohol abuse area, especially those working on or in alcohol dependency recovery. Alcoholism treatment and recovery services are, as described in this book, system responses to individuals who are experiencing personal and life problems associated with their drinking. Such services work with those who are most at risk individually for future life difficulties involving drinking, i.e., high-risk, targeted individuals. This book is not proposing that we abandon alcohol dependent persons nor fail to provide important and necessary services. However, we should be aware that even these services are created and maintained within, and contribute to, the same total community system which gives rise to problems in the first place. In short, we will never purposefully prevent nor substantially reduce alcohol-involved problems by simply treating heavy, dependent drinkers. Even if we are successful with the recovery of any individual dependent drinker, the system will continue to produce replacements. Treatment and recovery are not long-term prevention strategies for community level problems.

In like measure, the identification and targeting of groups within the community most at risk of alcohol problems (for example, young males under 25 years old have higher individual risk of acute alcohol problems like drinking and driving or violence) will result in the same failure. The community system will continue to produce replacements for any with whom we are individually successful. Thus alcohol problems will continue to occur, involving drinkers who are not dependent.

Second, abandoning a fondly held perspective is difficult enough but then to embrace a new world perspective which focuses on the community system rather than individuals is equally difficult. Little of what is done in alcohol problem prevention in most countries is based upon a complex adaptive community systems perspective. Few contemporary community prevention efforts are evaluated. However, most evaluated community prevention programs show little sustained effects.

Of course, one could take the position that popular (socially acceptable) and creative programs and policies are inherently good, and will be successful in the long run. Another conclusion, often advanced, is that we simply do not yet know enough important individual risk factors and when research provides such understanding, our prevention programs will become more successful. Both assumptions are quite nearsighted. Dynamic breaks with the past are necessary.

The lack of success in community prevention of alcohol-involved problems is inherent in the perspective (conceptual model) of the target group (catchment) approaches employed by almost all contemporary prevention practitioners throughout the world. The catchment approach is limited and is unlikely to ever produce long-term effects, i.e., sustained reductions in local alcohol problems. As we enter the 21st century, bold new perspectives and approaches will be required in most aspects of life. This book describes a way of thinking which can contribute to the fermentation of ideas and debate about what approaches to alcohol problem prevention should be advanced and encouraged, and which should be abandoned as old friends who can no longer serve us in the coming years.

References

Abel, E.L. & Sokol, R.J. (1991). A revised conservative estimate of the incidence of FAS and its economic impact. *Alcoholism: Clinical & Experimental Research*, **15**, 514–24.

Ackoff, R. & Emery, F.E. (1972). *On Purposeful Systems*. New York, NY: Aldine-Atherton.

Aitchison, J. & Brown, J.A.C. (1957). *The Lognormal Distribution*. Cambridge: Cambridge University Press.

Anda, R.F., Williamson, D.F. & Remington, P.L. (1988). Alcohol and fatal injuries among U.S. adults: findings from the NHANES I epidemiologic follow-up study. *Journal of the American Medical Association*, **260**, 2529–32.

Anderson, P. (1995). Alcohol and risk of physical harm. In *Alcohol and Public Policy: Evidence and Issues*, ed. H. Holder & G. Edwards, pp. 82–113. Oxford: Oxford University Press.

Anderson, P., Cremona, A., Paton, A., Turner, C., & Wallace, P. (1993). The risk of alcohol. *Addiction*, **88**, 1493–508.

Arthur, W.B. (1990). Positive feedbacks in the economy. *Scientific American*, February, 92–99.

Axelrod, R. (1984). *The Evolution of Cooperation*. New York, NY: Basic Books.

Axelrod, R. (1986). An evolutionary approach to norms. *American Political Science Review*, **80**, 1095–111.

Bales, F. (1946). Cultural differences in rates of alcoholism. *Quarterly Journal of Studies on Alcohol*, **6**, 480–99.

Beirness, D.J. (1984). Social drinkers estimates of blood alcohol concentrations: hypotheses and implications for safety. *Abstracts & Reviews in Alcohol & Driving*, **5**, 3–10.

Berry, B.J.L. (1968). Central place theory. In *Guide to Store Location Research*, ed. C. Kornblau, pp. 13–17. Reading, MA: Addison-Wesley Publishing Company.

Betancourt, R. & Gautschi, D. (1988). The economics of retail firms. *Managerial & Decision Economics*, **9**, 133–44.

Blane, H.W. (1974). Education and mass persuasion as preventive strategies. In *The Prevention of Alcohol Problems*, ed. R. Room & S. Sheffield, pp. 255–88. Berkeley, CA: The Social Research Group, University of California.

Blane, H. & Hewitt, L. (1977). *Mass Media, Public Education and Alcohol: A State of the Art Review*. Final report. National Institute on Alcohol Abuse and

Alcoholism. Springfield, VA: National Technical Information Service.

Blose, J.O. & Holder, H.D. (1987). Liquor-by-the-drink and alcohol-related traffic crashes: a natural experiment using time-series analysis. *Journal of Studies on Alcohol*, **48**, 52–60.

Boffetta, P. & Garfinkel, L. (1990). Alcohol drinking and mortality among men enrolled in an American Cancer Society prospective study. *Epidemiology*, **1**, 342–48.

Borkenstein, R.F. (1975). Problems of enforcement, adjudication and sanctioning. In *Alcohol, Drugs, and Traffic Safety*, ed. S. Israelstam & S. Lambert, pp. 655–62. Proceedings of the Sixth International Conference on Alcohol, Drugs, and Traffic Safety. Toronto: Addiction Research Foundation.

Box, G.E.P. & Jenkins, G.M. (1976). *Time Series Analysis: Forecasting and Control*. London: Holden-Day, Inc.

Brenner, H.M. (1975). Trends in alcohol consumption and associated illnesses: some effects of economic changes. *American Journal of Public Health*, **65**, 1279–92.

Brewer, G.O. (1983). Some costs and consequences of large-scale social systems modeling. *Behavioral Science*, **28**, 166–85.

Brown, M.M. & Wallace, P. (1980). *Alcoholic Beverage Taxation and Control Policies*, 4th edn. Ottawa: Brewers Association of Canada.

Bruun, K., Edwards, G., Lumio, M., Mäkelä, K., Pan, L., Popham, R.E., Room, R., Schmidt, W., Skog, O.J., Sulkunen, P., & Österberg, E. (1975). *Alcohol Control Policies in Public Health Perspective*. New Brunswick, NJ: Rutgers University Center of Alcohol Studies.

Bunce, R., Cameron, T., Collins, G., Morgan, P., Moser, J., & Room, R. (1981). California's alcohol experience: stable patterns and shifting responses. In *Alcohol, Society, and the State. 2. The Social History of Control Policy in Seven Countries*, ed. E. Single, P. Morgan, & J. deLint, pp. 159–97. Toronto: Addiction Research Foundation.

Caetano, R. (1987). Acculturation and attitudes toward appropriate drinking among U.S. Hispanics. *Alcohol & Alcoholism*, **22**, 427–33.

Caetano, R. (1988). A comparative analysis of drinking among Hispanics in the United States, Spaniards in Madrid, and Mexicans in Michoacan. In *Cultural Influences and Drinking Patterns: A Focus on Hispanic and Japanese Populations*, ed. T. Harford & L. Towle, pp. 237–311. Monograph. Rockville, MD: National Institute on Alcohol Abuse and Alcoholism.

Caetano, R. (1991). Findings from the 1984 National Survey of Alcohol Use Among U.S. Hispanics. In *Alcohol in America*, ed. W.B. Clark & M. Hilton, pp. 293–308. Albany, NY: State University of New York Press.

Caetano, R. (1995). *Prevalence, Violence, and Stability of Drinking Problems among Whites, Blacks, and Hispanics: 1984–1992*. Technical report. Berkeley, CA: Alcohol Research Group.

Caetano, R. & Kaskutas, L.A. (1996). Changes in drinking problems among Whites, Blacks, and Hispanics: 1984–1992. *Substance Use & Misuse*, **31**, 154–71.

Caetano, R. & Medina-Mora, M.E. (1988). Acculturation and drinking among people of Mexican descent in Mexico and the U.S. *Journal of Studies on Alcohol*, **49**, 462–71.

Cahalan, D. & Cisin, I.H. (1968). American drinking practices: summary of findings from a national probability sample. *Quarterly Journal of Studies on Alcohol*, **29**, 130–51.

Cahalan, D., Cisin, I.H., & Crossley, H.M. (1969). *American Drinking Practices.* New Brunswick, NJ: Rutgers University Center of Alcohol Studies.

Cahalan, D. & Room, R. (1972). Problem drinking among American men aged 21–59. *American Journal of Public Health,* **62,** 1473–82.

Cahalan, D. & Room, R. (1974). *Problem Drinking Among American Men.* New Brunswick, NJ: Rutgers University Center of Alcohol Studies.

Cameron, T. (1979). The impact of drinking-driving countermeasures: a review and evaluation. *Contemporary Drug Problems,* **8,** 495–565.

Casswell, S. (1995). Public discourse on alcohol: implications for public policy. In *Alcohol and Public Policy: Evidence and Issues,* ed. H.D. Holder & G. Edwards, pp. 190–211. New York, NY: Oxford University Press.

Casswell, S., Fang Zhang, J., & Wyllie, A. (1993). The importance of amount and location of drinking for the experience of alcohol-related problems. *Addiction,* **88,** 1527–34.

Casswell, S. & Gilmore, L. (1989). An evaluated community action project on alcohol. *Journal of Studies on Alcohol,* **50,** 339–46.

Casswell S., Gilmore, L., Maguire, V., & Ransom, R. (1989). Changes in public support for alcohol policies following a community-based campaign. *British Journal of Addiction,* **84,** 515–22.

Casti, J.L. (1992). *Reality Rules.* New York, NY: John Wiley and Sons.

Casti, J.L. (1994). *Complexification.* New York, NY: Harper Collins.

Cherpitel, C.J. (1988). Alcohol consumption and casualties: a comparison of two emergency room populations. *British Journal of Addiction,* **83,** 1299–1307.

Cherpitel, C.J. (1989). Breath analysis and self-reports as measures of alcohol-related emergency room admissions. *Journal of Studies on Alcohol,* **50,** 155–61.

Cherpitel, C.J. (1992). Epidemiology of alcohol-related trauma. *Alcohol, Health & Research World,* **16,** 191–96.

Cherpitel, C.J. (1993). Alcohol and injuries: a review of international emergency room studies. *Addiction,* **88,** 923–38.

Cherpitel, C.J. (1994). Alcohol and injuries resulting from violence: a review of emergency room studies. *Addiction,* **89,** 157–65.

Cherpitel, C.J. & Rosovsky, H. (1990). Alcohol consumption and casualties: a comparison of emergency room populations in the United States and Mexico. *Journal of Studies on Alcohol,* **51,** 319–428.

Churchman, C.W. (1979). *The Systems Approach and Its Enemies.* New York, NY: Basic Books.

Clark, W.B. (1991). Introduction. In *Alcohol in America: Drinking Practices and Problems,* ed. W.B. Clark & M.E. Hilton, pp. 1–16. Albany, NY: State University of New York Press.

Clark, W.B. & Hilton, M.E. (1991). *Alcohol in America: Drinking Practices and Problems.* Albany, NY: State University of New York Press.

Clark, W.B. & Midanik, L. (1982). Alcohol use and alcohol problems among U.S. adults: results of the 1979 national survey. In *Alcohol Consumption and Related Problems,* National Institute on Alcohol Abuse and Alcoholism, pp. 3–52. Alcohol and health monograph no. 1. Washington DC: Government Printing Office.

Clayton, A. (1986). Attitudes towards drinking and driving: their role in the effectiveness of countermeasures. *Alcohol, Drugs & Driving: Abstracts & Reviews,* **2,** 1–8.

Clements, D.W. (1978). Utility of linear models in retail geography. *Economic Geography*, **54**, 17–25.

Collins, J.J., Jr. (1981). Alcohol use and criminal behavior: an empirical, theoretical, and methodological overview. In *Drinking and Crime*, ed. J.J. Collins, pp. 288–316. New York, NY: Guilford.

Colon, I., Cutter, H.S.G., & Jones, W.C. (1982). Prediction of alcoholism from alcohol availability, alcohol consumption and demographic data. *Journal of Studies on Alcohol*, **43**, 1199–1213.

Comiti, V.P. (1990). The advertising of alcohol in France. *World Health Forum*, **11**, 242–45.

Cook, I., Dixon, R.T., Holder, H.D., Kennedy, F.D., Sawyer, L.L., Schlenger, W.E. & Williams, R.B. (1973). *Costs for Alternative Public Inebriation Services: Atlanta, Georgia*. Raleigh, NC: The Human Ecology Institute.

Cook, P.J. & Tauchen, G. (1982). The effect of liquor taxes on heavy drinking. *Bell Journal of Economics*, **13**, 379–90.

Cook, P.J. & Tauchen, G. (1984). The effect of minimum drinking age legislation on youthful auto fatalities, 1970–1977. *Journal of Legal Studies*, **13**, 169–90.

Corbett, K., Mora, J., & Ames, G. (1991). Drinking patterns and drinking-related problems of Mexican-American husbands and wives. *Journal of Studies on Alcohol*, **52**, 215–23.

Crouch, R.B. & Oglesby, S. (1978). Optimization of a few lot sizes to cover a range of requirements. *Journal of Operational Research Society*, **29**, 897–904.

Crow, E.L. & Shimizu, K. (eds.) (1988). *Lognormal Distributions*. New York, NY: Marcel Dekker, Inc.

Davies, P.C.W. (ed.) (1989). *The New Physics*. New York, NY: Cambridge University Press.

Devaney, R.L. (1989). *An Introduction to Chaotic Dynamical Systems*, 2nd edn. Redwood City, CA: Addison-Wesley Publishing Company.

Donnelly, P.G. (1978). Alcohol problems and sales in counties of Pennsylvania: a social area investigation. *Journal of Studies on Alcohol*, **39**, 848–58.

Douglas, R.R. (1990). Formulating alcohol policies for community recreation facilities: tactics and problems. In *Research, Action, and the Community: Experience in the Prevention of Alcohol and Other Drug Problems*, ed. N. Giesbrecht, P. Conley, R.W. Denniston, L. Gliksman, H. Holder, A. Pederson, R. Room, & M. Shain, pp. 61–67. Office of Substance Abuse Prevention monograph no. 4. Rockville, MD: Office for Substance Abuse Prevention.

Duffy, J.C. (1986). The distribution of alcohol consumption – 30 years on. *British Journal of Addiction*, **81**, 735–41.

Dunbar, J.A., Penttila, A., & Pikkarainen, J. (1987). Drinking and driving: success of random breath testing in Finland. *British Medical Journal*, **295**, 101–103.

Edwards, G., Anderson, P., Babor, T.F., Casswell, S., Ferrence, R., Giesbrecht, N., Godfrey, C., Holder, H.D., Lemmens, P., Mäkelä, K., Midanik, L.T., Norström, T., Österberg, E., Romelsjö, A., Room, R., Simpura, J., & Skog, O.J. (1994). *Alcohol Policy and the Public Good*. New York, NY: Oxford University Press.

Epstein, J.M. & Axtell, R.A. (1996). *Growing Artifical Societies: Social Science from the Bottom Up*. Washington DC: Brookings.

Fell, J. (1983). *Alcohol Involvement in U.S. Traffic Accidents: Where It Is Changing*. DOT HS 806–733, November. Washington DC: National

Highway Traffic Safety Administration, National Center for Statistics and Analysis.

Fillmore, K.M. (1987*a*). Prevalence, incidence and chronicity of drinking patterns and problems among men as a function of age: a longitudinal and cohort analysis. *British Journal of Addiction*, **82**, 77–83.

Fillmore, K.M. (1987*b*). Women's drinking across the adult life course as compared to men's. *British Journal of Addiction*, **82**, 801–11.

Fillmore, K.M. (1988). *Alcohol Use Across the Life Course: A Critical Review of 70 Years of International Longitudinal Research*. Toronto: Addiction Research Foundation.

Fillmore, K.M., Hartka, E., Johnstone, B.M., Leino, V., Motoyoshi, M., & Temple, M.T. (1991). The collaborative alcohol-related longitudinal project: a meta-analysis of life course variation in drinking. *British Journal of Addiction*, **86**, 1221–68.

Fisher, H., Simpson, R., & Kuper, B. (1987). Calculation of blood alcohol concentration (BAC) by sex, weight, number of drinks and time. *Canadian Journal of Public Health*, **78**, 300–304.

Forrester, J.W. (1969). *Urban Dynamics*. Cambridge, MA: MIT Press.

Frankel, B. & Whitehead, P.C. (1981). Drinking and damage: theoretical advances and implications for prevention. Monographs of the Rutgers Center for Alcohol Studies no. 14. New Brunswick, NJ: Rutgers University Center of Alcohol Studies.

Giesbrecht, N. (1993). Community action research since Scarborough: key issues facing us in 1992. In *Experiences with Community Action Projects: New Research in the Prevention of Alcohol and Other Drug Problems*, ed. T. Greenfield & R. Zimmerman, pp. 1–11. Rockville, MD: US Department of Health and Human Services, Public Health Service, Alcohol, Drug Abuse and Mental Health Administration.

Giesbrecht, N. & Pederson, A. (1991). Focusing on the drinking environment or the high-risk drinker in prevention projects: limitations and opportunities. In *Community Prevention Trials for Alcohol Problems: Methodological Issues*, ed. H.D. Holder & J.M. Howard, pp. 97–112. Westport, CT: Praeger Publishers.

Gliksman, L. (1986). Alcohol management policies for municipal recreation departments: an evaluation of the Thunder Bay model. In *Prevention and the Environment*, ed. N. Giesbrecht & A. Cox, pp. 198–204. Toronto: Addiction Research Foundation.

Gliksman, W., Douglas, R.R., Rylett, M., & Narbonne-Fortin, C. (1995). Reducing problems through municipal alcohol policies: The Canadian experience in Ontario. *Drugs: Education, Prevention & Policy*, **2**, 105–18.

Gliksman, L., Douglas, R.R., Thomson, M., Moffatt, K., Smythe, C., & Caverson, R. (1990). Promoting municipal alcohol policies: an evaluation of a campaign. *Contemporary Drug Problems*, **17**, 391–420.

Gliksman, L. & Rush, B.R. (1986). Alcohol availability, alcohol consumption and alcohol related damage. II. The role of sociodemographic factors. *Journal of Studies on Alcohol*, **47**, 11–18.

Glynn, R.J., Bouchard, G.R., LoCastro, J.S., & Laird, N.M. (1985). Aging and generational effects on drinking behaviors in men: results from the normative aging study. *American Journal of Public Health*, **75**, 1413–19.

Godfrey, C. (1988). Licensing and the demand for alcohol. *Applied Economics*, **20**, 1541–88.

Godfrey, C. (1990). Modeling demand. In *Preventing Alcohol and Tobacco*

Problems, vol. 1, ed. A. Maynard & P. Tether, pp. 35–53. Aldershot: Avebury.

Godfrey, C. (1991). Discussion of P. Cook's paper: the social costs of drinking. In *The Negative Social Consequences of Alcohol Use*, Norwegian Ministry of Health and Social Affairs in collaboration with the United Nations Office at Vienna, Centre for Social Development and Humanitarian Affairs, pp. 82–94. Oslo: Norwegian Ministry of Health and Social Affairs.

Godfrey, C. & Maynard, A. (1995). The economic evaluation of alcohol policies. In *Alcohol and Public Policy: Evidence and Issues*, ed. H.D. Holder & G. Edwards, pp. 238–59. New York, NY: Oxford University Press.

Grossman, M., Coate, D., & Arluck, G. (1987). Price sensitivity of alcoholic beverages in the United States: youth alcohol consumption. In *Control Issues in Alcohol Abuse Prevention: Strategies for States and Communities*, ed. H.D. Holder, pp. 169–98. Greenwich, CT: JAI Press.

Grube, J.W. & Wallack, L. (1994). Television beer advertising and drinking knowledge, beliefs, and intentions among schoolchildren. *American Journal of Public Health*, **84**, 254–59.

Gruenewald, P.J. (1988). Analytic models of alcohol consumption: dynamic models. Briefing paper no. 2. Berkeley, CA: Prevention Research Center.

Gruenewald, P.J., Madden, P., & Janes, K. (1992). Alcohol availability and the formal power and resources of state alcohol beverage control agencies. *Alcoholism: Clinical & Experimental Research*, **16**, 591–97.

Gruenewald, P.J., Ponicki, W.B., & Holder, H.D. (1993). The relationship of outlet densities to alcohol consumption: a time series cross-sectional analysis. *Alcoholism: Clinical & Experimental Research*, **17**, 38–47.

Gruenewald, P.J., Treno, A.J., Nephew, T.M., & Ponicki, W.R. (1995). Routine activities and alcohol use: constraints on outlet utilization. *Alcoholism: Clinical & Experimental Research*, **19**, 44–53.

Hallan, J.B. & Holder, H.D. (1986). Analysis of insurance benefit plans for alcoholism treatment through computer simulations. Parts 1 and II. *Computers in Psychiatry/Psychology*, **8**, no. 1, 12–15, no. 2, 12–15.

Hamilton, H.R., Goldstone, S.E., Milliman, J.W., Pugh, A.L., Roberts, E.R. & Zellner, A. (1969). *Systems Simulation for Regional Analysis: An Application to River-Basin Planning*. Cambridge, MA: MIT Press

Harford, T.C., Parker, D.A., Pautler, C., & Waltz, M. (1979). Relationship between the number of on-premises outlets and alcoholism. *Journal of Studies on Alcohol*, **40**, 1053–57.

Haskins, J.B. (1985). The role of mass media in alcohol and highway safety campaigns. *Journal of Studies on Alcohol*, **10**, 184–91.

Heien, D.M. & Pittman, D.J. (1989). The economic costs of alcohol abuse: an assessment of current methods and estimates. *Journal of Studies on Alcohol*, **50**, 567–79.

Herd, D. (1991). Drinking patterns in the Black population. In *Alcohol in America: Drinking Practices and Problems*, ed. W.B. Clark & M.E. Hilton, pp. 308–28. Albany, NY: State University of New York Press.

Hester, R.K. & Miller, W.R (ed.) (1989). *Handbook of Alcoholism Treatment Approaches: Effective Alternatives*. Elmsford, NY: Pergamon Press, Inc.

Hilton, M.E. (1986). Abstention in the general population of the U.S.A. *British Journal of Addiction*, **81**, 95–112.

Hilton, M.E. (1988). Trends in drinking problems and attitudes in the United States: 1979–1984. *British Journal of Addiction*, **83**, 1421–27.

Hilton, M.E. (1991). The presence of alcohol in four social situations: survey results from 1964 and 1984. In *Alcohol in America: Drinking Practices and Problems*, ed. W.B. Clark & M.E. Hilton, pp. 280–89. Albany, NY: State University of New York Press.

Hilton, M.E. & Clark, W.B. (1991). Changes in American drinking patterns and problems, 1967–1984. In *Alcohol in America: Drinking Practices and Problems*, ed. W.B. Clark & M.E. Hilton, pp. 105–20. Albany, NY: State University of New York Press.

Hingson, R. & Howland, J. (1987). Alcohol as a risk factor for injury or death resulting from accidental falls: a review of the literature. *Journal of Studies on Alcohol*, **48**, 212–19.

Hingson, R.W., Lederman, R.I. & Walsh, D.C. (1985). Employee drinking patterns and accidental injury: a study of four New England states. *Journal of Studies on Alcohol*, **46**, 298–303.

Hirschi, T. (1969). *Causes of Delinquency*. Berkeley, CA: Free Press.

Hoadley, J.F., Fuchs, B.C. & Holder, H.D. (1984). The effect of alcohol beverage restrictions on consumption: a 25–year longitudinal analysis. *American Journal of Drug & Alcohol Abuse*, **10**, 375–401.

Hochheimer, J. (1981). Reducing alcohol abuse: a critical review of educational strategies. In *Alcohol and Public Policy*, ed. M. Moore & D. Gerstein, pp. 286–335. Washington DC: National Academy Press.

Holder, H.D. (1987). Alcoholism treatment and potential health care cost saving. *Medical Care*, **25**, 52–71.

Holder, H.D. (1992). What is a community and what are implication for prevention trials for reducing alcohol problems? In *Community Prevention Trials for Alcohol Problems: methodological issues*, ed. H.D. Holder & J.M. Howard, pp. 15–34. Westport, CT: Praeger Publishers.

Holder, H.D. (1993). Prevention of alcohol-related accidents in the community. *Addiction*, **88**, 1003–12.

Holder, H.D. (1994). Public health approaches to the reduction of alcohol problems. *Substance Abuse*, **15**, 123–38.

Holder, H.D. (1996). Using computer models to predict prevention policy outcomes. *Alcohol Health & Research World*, **20** no. 4, 252–60.

Holder, H.D. (in press). Planning for alcohol problem prevention through complex systems modeling: results from *SimCom*. *Substance Use & Misuse*.

Holder, H.D. & Blose, J.O. (1983). Prevention of alcohol-related traffic problems: computer simulation of alternative strategies. *Journal of Safety Research*, **14**, 115–29.

Holder, H.D. & Blose, J.O. (1987). Reduction of community alcohol problems: computer simulation experiments in three counties. *Journal of Studies on Alcohol*, **48**, 124–35.

Holder, H.D. & Blose, J.O. (1988). Community planning and the prevention of alcohol involved traffic problems: an application of computer simulation technology. *Evaluation & Program Planning*, **11**, 267–77.

Holder, H.D. & Blose, J.O. (1992). The reduction of health care costs associated with alcoholism treatment: a 14–year longitudinal study. *Journal of Studies on Alcohol*, **53**, 293–302.

Holder, H.D. & Janes, K. (1989). Control of alcoholic beverages availability: state alcoholic beverage control systems having monopoly functions in the United States. In *State Monopolies and Alcohol Prevention*, ed. T. Kortteinen, pp. 355–460. Helsinki: The Social Research Institute of Alcohol Studies.

Holder, H.D., Janes, K., Mosher, J., Saltz, R., Spurr, S. & Wagenaar, A.C. (1993). Alcoholic beverage server liability and the reduction of alcohol-involved problems. *Journal of Studies on Alcohol,* **54,** 23–36.

Holder, H.D., Longabaugh, R., Miller, W.R. & Rubonis, A.V. (1991). The cost effectiveness of treatment for alcoholism: a first approximation. *Journal of Studies on Alcohol,* **52,** 517–40.

Holder, H.D., Saltz, R.F., Grube, J.W., Voas, R.B., Gruenewald, P.J. & Treno, A.J. (1997). A community prevention trial to reduce alcohol-involved accidental injury and death: overview. *Addiction,* **92,** Supplement 2, 8155–71.

Holder, H.D. & Wagenaar, A.C. (1990). Effects of the elimination of a state monopoly on distilled spirits' retail sales: a time-series analysis of Iowa. *British Journal of Addiction,* **85,** 1615–25.

Holder, H.D. & Wallack, L.M. (1986). Contemporary perspective for the prevention of alcohol problems: an empirically-derived model. *Journal of Public Health Policy,* **7,** 324–39.

Holland, J.H. (1975). *Adaptation in Natural and Artificial Systems.* Ann Arbor, MI: University of Michigan Press.

Holmila M. (ed.) (1997). *Community Prevention of Alcohol Problems.* London: MacMillan.

Holt, S., Stewart, I.C., Dixon, J.M.J., Elton, R.A., Taylor, T.V. & Little, K. (1980). Alcohol and the emergency service patient. *British Medical Journal,* **281,** 638–40.

Homel, R. (1988). *Policing and Punishing the Drinking Driver: A Study of General and Specific Deterrence.* New York, NY: Springer-Verlag.

Homel, R. (1993). Random breath testing in Australia: getting it to work according to specifications. *Addiction,* **88,** Supplement, S27–33.

Honkanen, R. (1993). Alcohol in home and leisure injuries. *Addiction,* **88,** 939–44.

Honkanen, R., Ertama, L., Kuosmanen, P., Linnoila, M., Alha, A. & Visuri, T. (1983). The role of alcohol in accidental falls. *Journal of Studies on Alcohol,* **44,** 231–45.

Howland, J. & Hingson, R. (1987). Alcohol as a risk factor for injuries or death due to fires or burns: review of the literature. *Public Health Reports,* **102,** 475–83.

Howland, J. & Hingson, R. (1988). Alcohol as a risk factor for drownings: a review of the literature. *Accident Analysis & Prevention,* **20,** 19–25.

Joksch, H C (1985). Review of the major risk factors. *Journal of Studies on Alcohol,* **10,** 47–53.

Johnson, P., Armor, D.J., Polich, S. & Stambul, H. (1977). *U.S. Adult Drinking Practices: Time Trends, Social Correlates and Sex Roles.* National Institute on Alcohol Abuse and Alcoholism, publication no. PB-294-044AS (ADM 281 76 0020). Springfield, VA: National Technical Information Service.

Jonah, B.A. & Wilson, R.J. (1983). Improving the effectiveness of drinking-driving enforcement through increased efficiency. *Accident Analysis & Prevention,* **15,** 463–81.

Kain, J. (1978). The use of computer simulation models for policy analysis. *Journal of Urban Analysis,* **5,** 175–89.

Kauffman, S.A. (1991). Antichaos and adaptation. *Scientific American,* August, 78–84.

Kauffman, S.A. (1993). *Origins of Order: Self-Organization and Selection in Evolution.* Oxford: Oxford University Press.

Kauffman, S.A. (1995). *At Home in the Universe.* New York, NY: Oxford University Press.

Kelly, J.G. (1990). Changing contexts and the field of community psychology. *American Journal of Community Psychology*, **18**, 769–92.

Kelly, J.G., Dassoff, N., Levin, I., Schreckengost, J., Stelzner, S.P. & Altman, B.E. (1988). *A Guide to Conducting Prevention Research in the Community: First Steps.* New York, NY: Haworth Press.

Kendell, R.E. (1984). The beneficial consequences of the United Kingdom's declining per capita consumption of alcohol in 1979–82. *Alcohol & Alcoholism*, **19**, 271–76.

Klatsky, A.L., Friedman, G.D. & Siegelaub, A.B. (1981). Alcohol and mortality: a ten-year Kaiser-Permanente experience. *Annals of Internal Medicine*, **95**, 139–45.

Klingemann, H., Takala, J.P. & Hunt, G. (ed.) (1992). *Cure, Care, or Control. Alcoholism Treatment in Sixteen Countries.* Albany, NY: State University of New York Press.

Klitzner, M., Gruenewald, P.J. & Bamberger, E. (1991). Cigarette advertising and adolescent experimentation with smoking. *British Journal of Addiction*, **86**, 287–98.

Klosterman, R.E. (1986). An assessment of three microcomputer software packages for planning analysis. *American Planning Association*, **52**, 199–202.

Knupfer, G. (1989). The prevalence of various social groups of eight different drinking patterns, from abstaining to frequent drunkenness: analysis of 10 U.S. surveys combined. *British Journal of Addiction*, **84**, 1305–18.

Knupfer, G. & Room, R. (1964). Age, sex and social class as factors in amount of drinking in a metropolitan community. *Social Problems*, **12**, 224–40.

Knupfer, G. & Room, R. (1970). Abstainers in a metropolitan community. *Quarterly Journal of Studies on Alcohol*, **31**, 108–31.

Kortteinen, T. (ed.) (1989). *State Monopolies and Alcohol Prevention.* Report no. 181. Helsinki: The Social Research Institute of Alcohol Studies.

Krige, D.G. (1966). A study of gold and uranium distribution patterns in the Klerksdorp Gold Field. *Geoxploration*, **4**, 45–53.

Lagerlof, E., Valverius, M. & Westerholm, P. (1984). Alcohol and fatal work accidents. *Journal of Occupational Accidents*, **6**, 1–3, 72.

Lakshmanan, T.R. & Hansen, W.G. (1965). A retail market potential model. *Journal of the American Institute of Planners*, **31**, 134–43.

Langendorf, R. (1985). Computers and decision making. *American Planning Association Journal*, **51**, 422–33.

Larsen, D.E. & Abu-Laban, B. (1968). Norm qualities and deviant drinking behavior. *Social Problems*, **15**, 441–50.

Larsen, R.I. (1969). A new mathematical model of air pollutant concentration averaging time and frequency. *Journal of the Air Pollution Control Association*, **19**, 24–30.

Law, A.M. & Kelton, W.D. (1982). *Simulation Modeling and Analysis.* New York, NY: McGraw-Hill.

Ledermann, S. (1964). *Alcool, Alcoolisme, Alcoolisation*, vol. II. Paris: Presses Universitarires de France.

Lemmons, P.H.H. (1995). Individual risk and population distribution of alcohol consumption. In *Alcohol and Public Policy: Evidence and Issues*, ed. H. Holder & G. Edwards, pp. 38–16. Oxford: Oxford University Press.

Lenke, L. (1990). *Alcohol and Criminal Violence: Time Series Analyses in a Comparative Perspective*. Stockholm: Almqvist and Wiksells.

Leung, S.F. & Phelps, C.E. (1993). My kingdom for a drink . . .? A review of estimates of the price sensitivity of demand for alcoholic beverages. In *Economics and the Prevention of Alcohol-Related Problems*, ed. M.E. Hilton & G. Bloss, pp. 1–32. Washington DC: National Institute on Alcohol Abuse and Alcoholism.

Levin, G., Roberts, E. & Hirsch, G.B. (1975). *The Persistent Poppy: A Computer-Aided Search for Heroin Policy*. Cambridge, MA: Ballinger.

Levy D. & Sheflin, N. (1983). New evidence on controlling alcohol use through price. *Journal of Studies on Alcohol*, **44**, 920–37.

Lewin, K. (1947). Frontiers in group dynamics. *Human Relations*, **1**, 2–38.

Linsky, A.S., Colby, J.P., Jr. & Straus, M.A. (1986). Drinking norms and alcohol-related problems in the United States. *Journal of Studies on Alcohol*, **47**, 384–93.

Linsky, A.S., Straus, M.A. & Colby, J.P., Jr. (1985). Stressful events, stressful conditions and alcohol problems in the United States: a partial test of Bale's theory. *Journal of Studies on Alcohol*, **46**, 72–80.

Loeb, G.F., Jr. (1978). Relationship of state law to per capita drinking. In *Drinking – Alcohol in American Society*, ed. J.A. Ewing & B.A. Rouse, pp. 219–39. Chicago, IL: Nelson-Hall.

MacDonald, S. & Whitehead, P.C. (1983). Availability of outlets and consumption of alcoholic beverages. *Journal of Drug Issues*, Fall, 477–86.

Maisto, S.A. & Rachal, J.V. (1980). Indications of the relationship among adolescent drinking practices, related behaviors, and drinking-age laws. In *Minimum-Drinking-Age Laws*, ed. H. Wechsler, pp. 155–76. Lexington, MA: Lexington Books.

Mäkelä, K. (1980). Differential effects of restricting the supply of alcohol: studies of a strike in Finnish liquor stores. *Journal of Drug Issues*, Winter, 131–44.

Mäkelä, K. (1991). Social and cultural preconditions of Alcoholics Anonymous (AA) and factors associated with the strength of AA. *British Journal of Addiction*, **86**, 1405–13.

Mäkelä, K., Österberg, E. & Sulkunen, P. (1991). Drinking in Finland: increasing alcohol availability in a monopoly state. In *Alcohol, Society and the State. 2. The History of Control Policy in Seven Countries*, ed. E. Single, P. Morgan, & J. deLint, pp. 31–60. Toronto: Addiction Research Foundation.

Mäkelä, K., Room, R., Single, E., Sulkunen, P. & Walsh, B. (1981). *Alcohol, Society and the State. 1. A Comparative Study of Alcohol Control*. Toronto: Addiction Research Foundation.

Markides, K.S., Krause, N. & Mendes de Leon, C.F. (1988). Acculturation and alcohol consumption among Mexican Americans: a three-generation study. *American Journal of Public Health*, **78**, 1178–81.

Markin, R.J., Jr. (1974). *Consumer Behavior. A Cognitive Orientation*. New York, NY: MacMillan.

Marshall, M. & Marshall, L.B. (1990). *Silent Voices Speak. Women and Prohibition in Truk*. Belmont, CA: Wadsworth Publishing Company.

Matlins, S.M. (1976). *A Study in the Actual Effects of Alcoholic Beverage Control Laws*, vol. 1 & vol. 2. National Institute on Alcohol Abuse and Alcoholism report. Washington DC: Medicine in the Public Interest.

Matsueda, R.L. (1982). Testing control theory and differential association: A causal modeling approach. *American Sociological Review*, **47**, 489–504.

Matsueda, R.L. & Heimer, K. (1987). Race, family structure, and deliquency: a test of differential association and social control theories. *American Sociological Review*, **52**, 826–40.

McCleary, R., Hay, R.A., McDowall, D. & Meidinger, E.E. (1980). *Applied Time Series Analysis for the Social Sciences*. Beverly Hills & London: Sage Publications.

McCrady, B.S. & Miller, W.R. (ed.) (1993). *Research on Alcoholics Anonymous: Opportunities and Alternatives*. New Brunswick, NJ: Rutgers University Center of Alcohol Studies.

McLean, S. (1976). A comparison of the lognormal and transition models of wastage. *Statistician*, **24**, 281–94.

Meier, R.F. (1982). Perspectives on the concept of social control. *Annual Review of Sociology*, **8**, 35–55.

Miller, T., Pindus, N.M., Douglass, J.B. & Rossman, S.B. (1995). *Databook on Nonfatal Injury: Incidence, Costs, and Consequences*. Washington DC: The Urban Institute Press.

Miller, W.R., Heather, N. & Hall, W. (1991). Calculating standard drink units: international comparisons. *British Journal of Addiction*, **86**, 43–7.

Mitroff, I. & Sagasti, F. (1973). Epistomology as general systems theory: an approach to the design of complex decision-making experiments. *Philosophy of the Social Services*, **3**, 117–34.

Moore, M. & Gerstein, D. (eds.) (1981). *Alcohol and Public Policy: Beyond the Shadow of Prohibition*. Washington DC: National Academy Press.

Mosher, J.F. (1983). Server intervention: a new approach for preventing drinking driving. *Accident Analysis & Prevention*, **15**, 483–97.

Moskowitz, J.M. (1989). The primary prevention of alcohol problems: a critical review of the research literature. *Journal of Studies on Alcohol*, **50**, 54–88.

Mouden, J.V. & Russell, A. (1994). 'Is it MADD trying to rate the states?' – a citizen activist approach to DWI prevention. *Alcohol, Drugs & Driving*, **10**, 317–26.

National Institute on Drug Abuse (1988). *National Household Survey on Drug Abuse: Main Findings 1985*. Rockville, MD: US Deptartment of Health and Human Services, Public Health Service, Alcohol, Drug Abuse and Mental Health Administration.

National Institute on Drug Abuse (1990). *National Household Survey on Drug Abuse: Main Findings 1988*. Rockville, MD: US Deptartment of Health and Human Services, Public Health Service, Alcohol, Drug Abuse and Mental Health Administration.

Nelson, J. (1988). *The Economic and Legal Determinants of Alcoholic Beverage Consumption in the US: A Bayesian Approach*. University Park, PA: Department of Economics, Pennsylvania State University.

Nicolis, G. & Prigogine, I. (1989). *Exploring Complexity*. New York, NY: W.H. Freeman.

Nooteboom, B., Kleijweg, A. & Thurik, A.R. (1988). Normal costs and demand effects in price setting. *European Economic Review*, **32**, 999–1011.

Norström, T. (1987). The impact of per capita consumption on Swedish cirrhosis mortality. *British Journal of Addiction*, **82**, 67–75.

Norström, T. (1988). Alcohol and suicide in Scandinavia. *British Journal of Addiction*, **83**, 553–59.

O'Malley, P.M. & Wagenaar, A.C. (1991). Effects of minimum drinking age laws on alcohol use, related behaviors, and traffic crash involvement among

American youth: 1976–1987. *Journal of Studies on Alcohol*, **52**, 478–91.

Ornstein, S.I. & Hanssens, D.M. (1981). *Alcohol Control Laws, Consumer Welfare, and the Demand for Distilled Spirits and Beer*. Working paper series no. 102. Los Angeles, CA: Graduate School of Management, University of California.

Ornstein, S.I. & Hanssens, D.M. (1985). Alcohol control laws and the consumption of distilled spirits and beer. *Journal of Consumer Research*, **12**, 200–13.

Ornstein, S.I. & Levy, D. (1983). Price and income elasticities and the demand for alcoholic beverages. In *Recent Developments in Alcoholism*, vol. 1, ed. M. Galanter, pp. 303–45. New York, NY: Plenum.

Österberg, E. (1991). Current approaches to limit alcohol abuse and the negative consequences of use: a comparative overview of available options and an assessment of proven effectiveness. In *The Negative Social Consequences of Alcohol Use*, ed. O. Aasland, pp. 266–69. Oslo: Norwegian Ministry of Health and Social Affairs.

Österberg, E. (1995). Do alcohol prices affect consumption and related problems? In *Alcohol and Public Policy: Evidence and Issues*, ed. H. Holder & G. Edwards, pp. 143 63. Oxford & New York, NY: Oxford University Press.

Parker, D.A., Wolz, M.W. & Harford, T.C. (1978). The prevention of alcoholism: an empirical report on the effects of outlet availability. *Alcoholism: Clinical & Experimental Research*, **2**, 339–43.

Parker, R.N. (1995). Bringing "booze" back in: the relationship between alcohol and homicide. *Journal of Research in Crime & Delinquency*, **32**, 3–38.

Parker, R.N. & Rebhun, L.A. (1995). *Alcohol and Homicide: A Deadly Combination of Two American Traditions*. Albany, NY: State University of New York Press.

Partanen, J. (1990). Alcohol in culture and social life. *Alcologia*, **2**, 23–32.

Partanen, J. & Montonen, M. (1988). *Alcohol and the Mass Media*. EURO Reports and Studies no. 108. Copenhagen: World Health Organization, Regional Office for Europe.

Payne, J.A. (1982). *Introduction to Simulation: Programming Techniques and Methods of Analysis*. New York, NY: McGraw Hill.

Peltzman, S. (1975). The effects of automobile safety legislation. *Journal of Political Economy*, **83**, 667–725.

Perelson, A.S. & Kauffman, S.A. (eds.) (1990). *Molecular Evolution on Rugged Landscapes: Proteins, RNA, and the Immune System*. Santa Fe Institute Studies in the Sciences of Complexity, Proceedings vol. 9. Redwood City, CA: Addison-Wesley Publishing Company.

Pindyck, R S & Rubinfeld, D.L. (1989). *Microeconomics*. New York, NY: MacMillan.

Pittman, D.J. (1967). International overview: social and cultural factors in drinking patterns, pathological and nonpathological. In *Alcoholism*, ed. D.J. Pittman, pp. 3–20. New York, NY: Harper and Row Publications, Inc.

Pittman, D.J. & Snyder, C.R. (1962). *Society, Culture, and Drinking Patterns*. New York, NY: John Wiley and Sons.

Pugh, A.L., III. (1973). *Dynamo II User's Manual*, 4th edn. Cambridge, MA: MIT Press.

Rabow, J. & Watts, R.K. (1982). Alcohol availability, alcoholic beverage sales and alcohol-related problems. *Journal of Studies on Alcohol*, **44**, 767–801.

Reed, D. (1981). Reducing the costs of drinking and driving. In *Alcohol and Public*

Policy, ed. M. Moore & D. Gerstein, pp. 336–87. Washington DC: National Academy Press.

Rice, D.P., Kelman, S. & Miller, L.S. (1990). *The Economic Costs of Alcohol and Drug Abuse and Mental Illness, 1985*. San Francisco, CA: San Francisco Institute for Health and Aging.

Roman, P.M. (ed.) (1990). *Alcohol Problem Intervention in the Workplace*: *Employee Assistance Programs and Strategic Alternatives*. New York, NY: Quorum Books.

Room, R. (1972). Drinking patterns in large U.S. cities – a comparison of San Francisco and national samples. *Quarterly Journal of Studies on Alcohol*, Supplement no. 6, 28–57.

Room, R. (1983). Region and urbanization as factors in drinking practices and problems. In *The Pathogenesis of Alcoholism*: *Psychological Factors*, The Biology of Alcoholism, vol. 6, ed. B. Kissin & H. Begleiter, pp. 555–604. New York, NY: Plenum.

Room, R. (1989). Cultural changes in drinking and trends in alcohol problem indicators: recent U.S. experience. In *Prevention and Control/Realities and Aspirations*, ed. R. Waahlberg, pp. 820–31. Proceedings of the 35th International Congress on Alcoholism and Drug Dependence. Oslo: National Directorate for the Prevention of Alcohol and Drug Problems.

Room, R. (1991). Cultural changes in drinking and trends in alcohol problems indicators: recent U.S. experience. In *Alcohol in America*, ed. W.G. Clark & M.E. Hilton, pp. 149–62. Albany, NY: State University of New York Press.

Rosenberg, N., Laessig, R. & Rawlings, R.R. (1974). Alcohol, age, and fatal traffic accidents. *Quarterly Journal of Studies on Alcohol*, **35**, 473–89.

Ross, H.L. (1982). *Deterring the Drinking Driver*: *Legal Policy and Social Control*. Lexington, MA: D.C. Heath and Company.

Ross, H.L. (1983). Limitations on deterring the drinking driver. *Abstracts & Reviews on Alcohol & Driving*, **4**, 3–8.

Ross, H.L. (1985). Deterring drunken driving: an analysis of current efforts. *Journal of Studies on Alcohol*, Supplement no. 10, 122–28.

Rossow, I. (1993). Suicide, alcohol, and divorce: aspects of gender and family integration. *Addiction*, **88**, 1659–65.

Rush, R. & Gliksman, L. (1986). The distribution of consumption approach to the prevention of alcohol-related damage: an overview of relevant research and current issues. *Advances in Alcohol & Substance Abuse*, **5**, 9–32.

Rush, B.R., Steinberg, M. & Brook, R. (1986). The relationships among alcohol availability, alcohol consumption and alcohol-related damage in the Province of Ontario and the State of Michigan 1955–1982. *Advances in Alcohol & Substance Abuse*, **5**, 33–45.

Russ, N.W., Harwood, M.K. & Geller S. (1986). Estimating alcohol impairment in the field: implications for drunken driving. *Journal of Studies on Alcohol*, **47**, 237–40.

Rydell, C. & Everingham, S. (1994). *Controlling Cocaine*: *Supply Versus Demand Programs*. Office of National Drug Control Policy, U.S. Army report. Santa Monica, CA: RAND.

Saffer, H. (1993). Advertising under the influence. In *Economics and the Prevention of Alcohol-Related Problems*, ed. M.E. Hilton & G. Bloss, pp. 125–40. Washington DC: National Institute on Alcohol Abuse and Alcoholism.

Saffer, H. & Grossman, M. (1987). Beer taxes, the legal drinking age, and youth motor vehicle fatalities. *Journal of Legal Studies*, **16**, 351–74.

Saltz, R.F., Gruenewald, P.J. & Hennessy, M. (1992). Candidate alcohol problems and implications for measurement: general alcohol problems, outcome measures, instrumentation, and surrogates. In *Community Prevention Trials for Alcohol Problems: Methodological Issues*, ed. H.D. Holder & J.M. Howard, pp. 35–56. Westport, CT: Praeger Publishers.

Sarason, S. (1974). *The Psychological Sense of Community: Prospects for a Community Psychology*. San Francisco, CA: Jossey-Bass, Inc.

Schmidt, W. & Kornaczewski, A. (1975). The effect of lowering the legal drinking age in Ontario and on alcohol-related motor vehicle accidents In *Alcohol, Drugs, and Traffic Safety*, ed. S. Israelstam & S. Lambert, pp. 763–70. Proceedings of the Sixth International Conference on Alcohol, Drugs, and Traffic Safety. Toronto: Addiction Research Foundation.

Seal, H.L. (1969). *Stochastic Theory of a Risk Business*. New York, NY: John Wiley and Sons.

Seidman, E. (1988). Back to the future, community psychology: unfolding a theory of social intervention. *American Journal of Community Psychology*, **16**, 3–24.

Simpura, J. (ed.) (1987). *Finnish Drinking Habits. Results from Surveys Held in 1968, 1976 and 1984*. Helsinki: Finnish Foundation for Alcohol Studies.

Simpura, J. (1995). Trends in alcohol consumption and drinking patterns: lessons from world-wide development. In *Alcohol and Public Policy: Evidence and Issues*, ed. H.D. Holder & G. Edwards, pp. 9–37. New York, NY: Oxford University Press.

Skog, O.J. (1980). Social interaction and the distribution of alcohol consumption. *Journal of Drug Issues*, **10**, 71–92.

Skog, O.J. (1982). *The Distribution of Alcohol Consumption. Part I. A Critical Discussion of the Ledermann Model*. SIFA mimeographed series no. 64. Oslo: National Institute for Alcohol Research.

Skog, O.J. (1985). The collectivity of drinking cultures: a theory of the distribution of alcohol consumption. *British Journal of Addiction*, **80**, 83–99.

Skog, O.J. (1986). An analysis of divergent trends in alcohol consumption and economic development. *Journal of Studies on Alcohol*, **47**, 19–25.

Skog, O.J. & Elekes, S. (1993). Alcohol and the 1950–90 Hungarian suicide trend. Is there a causal connection? *Acta Sociologica*, **36**, 33–46.

Smart, R.G. (1977). Changes in alcoholic beverage sales after reductions in the legal drinking age. *American Journal of Drug & Alcohol Abuse*, **4**, 101–108.

Smart, R.G. (1988). Does alcohol advertising affect overall consumption? A review of empirical studies. *Journal of Studies on Alcohol*, **49**, 314–23.

Smart, R.G. & Fejer, D. (1975). Six years of cross-sectional surveys of student drug use in Toronto. *Bulletin on Narcotics*, **27**(2), 11–22.

Smith, G.S. & Kraus, J.F. (1988). Alcohol and residential, recreational and occupational injuries: a review of the epidemiological evidence. *Annual Review of Public Health*, **9**, 99–121.

Stockwell, R., Lange, E. & Rydon, P. (1993). High risk drinking settings: the association of serving and promotional practices with harmful drinking. *Addiction*, **88**, 1519–26.

Stonier, R.J. & Yu, X.H. (1994). *Complex Systems: Mechanism of Adaptation*. Amsterdam: IOS Press.

Stout, R.L. (1992). Prevention experiments in the context of on-going community process: opportunities or obstacles for research. In *Community Prevention*

Trials for Alcohol Problems: Methodological Issues, ed. H.D. Holder & J.M. Howard, pp. 121–33. Westport, CT: Praeger Publishers.

Summers, L.G. & Harris, D.H. (1978). *The General Deterrence of Driving While Intoxicated. Vol. I: System Analysis and Computer-Based Simulation*. NTIS no. PB-288 112. Washington DC; US Department of Transportation, US Department of Commerce.

Sutherland, E.H. (1947). *Principles of Criminology*, 4th edn. Philadelphia, PA: Lippincott.

Tan, E.S., Lemmens, P.H.H.M. & Koning, A.J. (1990). Regularity in alcohol distributions: implications for the collective nature of drinking behavior. *British Journal of Addiction*, **85**, 745–50.

Teplin, L.A., Abram, K.M. & Michaels, S.K. (1989). Blood alcohol level among emergency room patients: a multivariate analysis. *Journal of Studies on Alcohol*, **50**, 441–47.

Thorsen, T. (1990). *Hundrede ars alkoholmisbrug*. [*One Hundred Years of Alcohol Abuse: Alcohol Consumption and Alcohol Problems in Denmark.*] Copenhagen: Alkohol- og Narkotikartadet.

Tiao, G.C. & Box, G.E.P. (1981). Modeling multiple time series with application. *Journal of the American Statistical Association*, **76**, 802–16.

Treno, A.J., Parker, R.N. & Holder, H.D. (1993). Understanding U.S. alcohol consumption with social and economic factors: a multivariate series analysis, 1950–1986. *Journal of Studies on Alcohol*, **54**, 146–56.

United States General Accounting Office. (1987). *Drinking-Age Law: An Evaluation Synthesis of Their Impact on Highway Safety*. GAO/PEMD 87–10, March. Washington DC: US General Accounting Office.

Voas, R.B. & Hause, J.M. (1987). Deterring the drinking driver: the Stockton experience. *Accident Analysis & Prevention*, **19**, 81–90.

Wagenaar, A.C. (1983). *Alcohol, Young Drivers, and Traffic Accidents*. Lexington, MA: Lexington Books.

Wagenaar, A.C. (1986). Preventing highway crashes by raising the legal minimum age for drinking: the Michigan experience six years later. *Journal of Safety Research*, **17**, 101–109.

Wagenaar, A.C. & Holder, H.D. (1991). Effects of alcoholic beverage server liability on traffic crash injuries. *Alcoholism: Clinical & Experimental Research*, **15**, 942–47.

Wagenaar, A.C. & Holder, H.D. (1995). Changes in alcohol consumption resulting from the elimination of retail wine monopolies: results from five U.S. states. *Journal of Studies on Alcohol*, **56**, 566–72.

Wagenaar, A.C. & Wolfson, M. (1994). Enforcement of the legal minimum drinking age in the United States. *Journal of Public Health Policy*, **15**, 37–53.

Waldrup, M.M. (1992). *Complexity: The Emerging Science at the Edge of Order and Chaos*. New York, NY: Simon and Schuster.

Wallack, L.M. (1981). Mass media campaigns: the odds against finding behavior change. *Health Education Quarterly*, **8**, 209–60.

Wallack, L., Grube, J.W., Madden, P.A. & Breed, W. (1990). Portrayals of alcohol on prime-time television. *Journal of Studies on Alcohol*, **51**, 428–37.

Watts, R.K. & Rabow, J. (1983). Alcohol availability and alcohol-related problems in 213 California cities. *Alcoholism: Clinical & Experimental Research*, **7**, 47–58.

Wechsler, H., Demone, H.W. & Gottlieb, M.A. (1978). Drinking patterns of

Greater Boston adults – subgroup differences on the QFV Index. *Journal of Studies on Alcohol*, **39**, 1158–65.

Wechsler, H., Kasey, E.H., Thum, D. & Demone, H.W. (1969). Alcohol level and home accidents. *Public Health Reports*, **84**, 1043–50.

Whitehead, J.T. & Lab, S.P. (1989). A meta-analysis of juvenile correctional treatment. *Journal of Research in Crime & Delinquency*, **26**, 276–95.

Whitehead, P.C. (1975). DWI programs: doing what's in or doing what's indicated? *Journal of Safety Research*, **7**, 127–34.

Whitehead, P.C., Craig, S., Langford, N., MacArthur C., Stanton, B. & Ferrence, R.G. (1975). Collision behavior of young drivers: impact of the change in the age of majority. *Journal of Studies on Alcohol*, **36**, 1208–23.

Wilde, G.J.S. (1982). The theory of risk homeostasis: implications for safety and health. *Risk Analysis*, **2**, 209–25.

Williams, A.F., Rich, R.F., Zador, P.L. & Robertson, L.S. (1975). The legal minimum drinking age and fatal motor vehicle crashes. *The Journal of Legal Studies*, **4**, 219–39.

Wittman, F.D. & Hilton, M.E. (1987). Uses of planning and zoning ordinances to regulate alcohol outlets in California cities. In *Control Issues in Alcohol Abuse Prevention: Strategies for States and Communities*, Supplement no. 1, ed. H. Holder, pp. 337–66. Greenwich, CT: JAI Press.

Wolfgang, M.E. (1958). *Patterns in Criminal Homicide*. Philadelphia, PA: University of Pennsylvania Press.

Wolfson, M., Toomey, T., Murray, D., Forster, J., Short, B., & Wagenaar, A. (1996). Alcohol outlet policies and practices concerning sales to underage people. *Addiction*, **91**, 589–602.

Zador, P., Lund, A., Fields, M. & Weinburg, K. (1988). *Fatal Crash Involvement and Laws Against Alcohol-impaired Driving*. Washington DC: Insurance Institute for Highway Safety.

Zobeck, T. (1986). *Trends in Alcohol-Related Fatal Traffic Accidents, United States: 1977–1984*. Surveillance Report no. 1. Alcohol Epidemiologic Data System. Washington DC: CSR, Inc.

Zobeck, T.S., Elliott, S.D., Grant, B.F. & Bertolucci, M.A. (1991). *Trends in Alcohol-Related Fatal Traffic Crashes, United States: 1977–1988*. Surveillance Report no. 17. Alcohol Epidemiologic Data System. Washington DC: CSR, Inc.

Index

Note: page numbers in *italics* refer to figures and tables